NUMEROLOGY

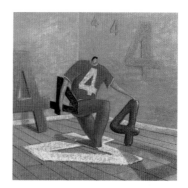

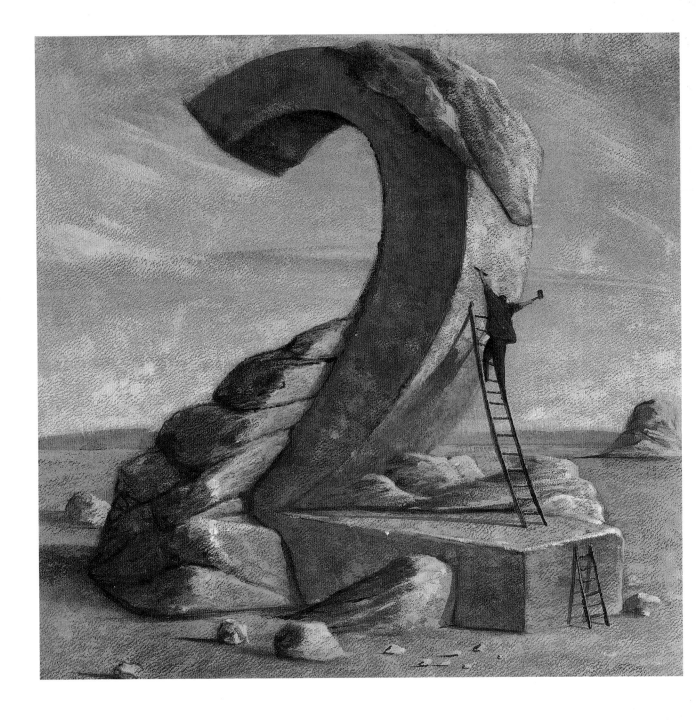

NUMEROLOGY

USING THE POWER OF NUMBERS TO DISCOVER AND SHAPE YOUR DESTINY

COLIN-M BAKER

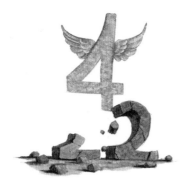

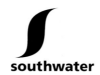

southwater

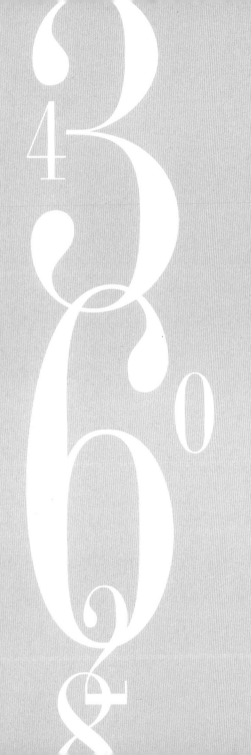

This edition is published by Southwater, an imprint of Anness Publishing Ltd, Hermes House, 88–89 Blackfriars Road, London SE1 8HA; tel. 020 7401 2077; fax 020 7633 9499

www.southwaterbooks.com;
www.annesspublishing.com

If you like the images in this book and would like to investigate using them for publishing, promotions or advertising, please visit our website www.practicalpictures.com for more information.

UK agent: The Manning Partnership Ltd; tel. 01225 478444; fax 01225 478440; sales@manning-partnership.co.uk
UK distributor: Grantham Book Services Ltd; tel. 01476 541080; fax 01476 541061; orders@gbs.tbs-ltd.co.uk
North American agent/distributor: National Book Network; tel. 301 459 3366; fax 301 429 5746; www.nbnbooks.com
Australian agent/distributor: Pan Macmillan Australia; tel. 1300 135 113; fax 1300 135 103; customer.service@macmillan.com.au
New Zealand agent/distributor: David Bateman Ltd; tel. (09) 415 7664; fax (09) 415 8892

Publisher: Joanna Lorenz
Managing Editor: Helen Sudell
Project Editor: Simona Hill
Copy Editor: Jenny Barrett
Designer: Louise Clements
Reader: Hayley Kerr
Production: Joanna King

ETHICAL TRADING POLICY

Because of our ongoing ecological investment programme, you, as our customer, can have the pleasure and reassurance of knowing that a tree is being cultivated on your behalf to naturally replace the materials used to make the book you are holding. For further information about this scheme, go to www.annesspublishing.com/trees

AUTHOR'S ACKNOWLEDGEMENTS

My thanks go to Claudine Aegerter, Principal of the Connaissance School of Numerology, whose knowledge and insight inspired me to take up the subject. I am also totally indebted to friend and colleague Berenice Benjelloun, fellow numerologist and teacher, who beavered away for long hours putting the book on disk. My gratitude also goes to her husband, Olly, who must have wondered at times if I had moved in, but who always made me feel completely welcome. Finally, thanks to my publishers for their patience.

AUTHOR'S NOTE

The letter-to-number translation system used in this book is based on the 26 letters of the English alphabet. Different alphabets and spellings will inevitably produce different aggregations of numbers. Remember though that spirit is universal, and the soul of each country, expressed through its language, speaks of its own part in the evolution of human consciousness. So try it both ways, first translate a name or word using the English system, then do it again using your own alphabet/spelling and ponder on the different results, and what they mean; discover the underlying unity that lies behind both systems.

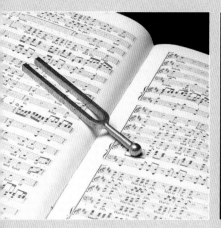
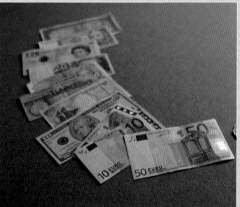
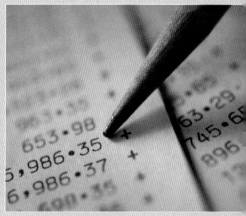

contents

introduction

Numerology is the art of understanding life by studying the symbolic value of numbers and the relationships between them.

Over thousands of years, each of the whole numbers one to nine has become associated with a set of meanings and characteristics. Numerology takes these numbers beyond their use in everyday calculations. It explores their significance as symbols of the energies of the universe, relating their symbolic value to important numbers in our lives.

Numerology addresses the spiritual dimension of life. It is associated with several different major religious traditions as well as esoteric studies such as tarot and astrology. It gives us a way of expressing symbolically our development through progressively higher stages of consciousness within the many cycles of our lives. What our numbers reveal can clarify how we perceive ourselves, others, and our environment. If we understand our nature better and learn to recognize the cyclical trends in our world then we can work with our innate qualities and the patterns of our lives harmoniously.

Many people regard numerology as a science, with its own internal logic and structured, systematic approach. How numbers are read and used symbolically reflects our ability to interpret them: numerology relies on instinct and intuition as well as a sound understanding of the principles involved.

Neither the meanings attached to the numbers nor the way we work with them are fixed. Nevertheless, if you trust them sufficiently, the numbers can serve as guideposts, pointing you to an understanding of yourself, and showing you how best to take your life's journey in a positive direction. Even if you feel sceptical at first, you too have the potential to access the meaning of numbers and understand them in a way that makes sense to you if you approach them with an open heart and an open mind. The more you explore the numbers and their meanings the greater will be your sensitivity to the energy flowing through them.

Numerology is a discipline that can be approached at many levels. This book will help you to take your first steps into this complex and fascinating subject – use it as a springboard for your own creative and spiritual explorations as you become attuned to the energy of the universe.

RIGHT AND OPPOSITE: *Our lives are filled with significant numbers. In numerology numbers are like a signpost helping us to fulfil our potential.*

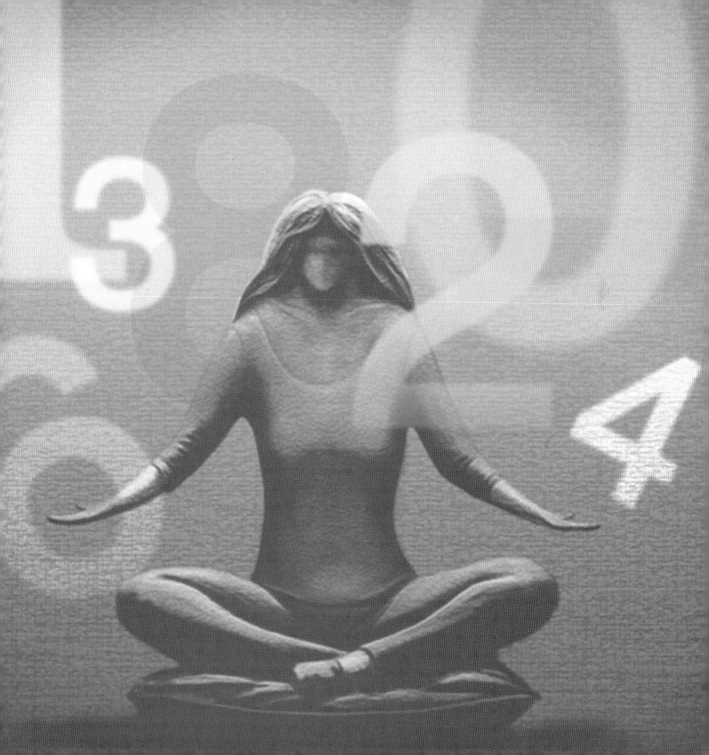

a brief history of numerology

It is difficult to say precisely when or where numerology started. Many cultures and religions all over the world have either devised their own system of working with numbers in a symbolic way, or borrowed from and expanded on existing ones. All of them have been used to explain and gain a deeper understanding of who we are and the world we live in, and a few have developed ways of working with numbers that have survived to this day.

ORIGINS

Chaldean numerology is accepted by many as the most ancient tradition – some claim that it dates back more than 400,000 years. With a focus on the personality rather than the soul, and on prediction rather than an understanding of the world, it has its practitioners to this day.

Cultures and religions through the ages have used numbers in a symbolic way

NUMEROLOGY FAR AND WIDE

Various forms of numerology have been practised in civilizations around the world: the Hindu Brahmins of India were major contributors to the history of numerology; there are Oriental systems of numbers that are still in use in the East; and the Mayan calendar, in which certain key dates are

associated with major changes, still commands wide attention. Numerology's most refined expression is found in the Tree of Life of the Judaic Kabbalistic tradition, with its uniquely linked alphabet, symbols and sounds, and there are also clear parallels to be drawn between this system and the Tarot, the earliest evidence of which is found during the Middle Ages in Europe.

NUMEROLOGY IN THE WEST

By far the most influential figure in Western numerology is Pythagoras (c.582–507BC). He travelled extensively in Europe and Asia and was strongly influenced by those he met, including the followers of the Persian prophet Zoroaster and Brahmin priests in India. He was also initiated into various mystery schools and the secret teachings of the Chaldeans of Babylon. Pythagoras eventually established his own school of mysteries in Italy. Central to its work were mathematics, music, and astronomy, which then included astrology. All three had the principle of number as their basis. Indeed, a fundamental concept of Pythagoreanism was that the universe was essentially a manifestation of mathematical relationships, a

ABOVE: *The numbered cards in the major arcana of the Tarot show progressions of development comparable to those found in numerology.* RIGHT: *For Pythagoras, harmony in music came from the mathematical relationships between sound vibrations.*

harmonious whole in which everything had its own vibration or sound tone that could be expressed in numbers and related to each other through geometry. His belief in reincarnation was consistent with the idea that life is cyclical, and that we can develop as individuals as a result of learning from what has occurred in previous cycles. Although Pythagoras used numbers to predict future events, this was not his primary motivation in working with them.

Western numerology has evolved and adapted slowly since Pythagoras, with shifts in emphasis and use rather than real landmark changes. For example, with the fascination for science that arose in the 19th century, discoveries involving light, magnetism, and electricity helped to popularize the theory that numbers related to energy patterns of vibrations. In modern times the person who has most influenced the way we view numerology is Sepharial, who studied a range of occult sciences in the late 19th and early 20th centuries. In his classic two-volume work, *The Kabalah of Numbers*, he explored the relationships between numerology and astrology, numbers and names, and numbers and nature (especially colour, sound, planetary motion and cycles). Intriguingly, he also harnessed the powers of astrology and numerology to predict – with some success – the movement of stocks and shares and the results of horse races!

Through the centuries numerology has been used in many contexts and for many purposes. It has been used to understand nature, to make predictions, and to explore the hidden meanings of the Bible. Its main use today, as a tool to give us insight into our personal lives, is consistent with our increasing focus on personal and spiritual development.

21 DECEMBER 2012: *End of an Age*

The ancient Mayans of Mesoamerica developed a complex and accurate calendar, based on astronomical observations and mathematical calculations. The date 13.0.0.0.0 on the Mayan calendar, corresponding to 21 December 2012, represents the end of a cycle lasting 5125 years. Unlike our calendar, which counts the years that have elapsed since a critical event (the birth of Christ), the Mayan calendar was reckoned backwards from a cataclysmic event which they predicted would occur in the future, and which would herald the start of a new era. Their understanding of astronomy was so sophisticated that they could calculate this date accurately, 2300 years in advance. At this time the winter solstice sun would be in a rare conjunction with the crossing point of the Milky Way's equator – a significant event in their mythology.

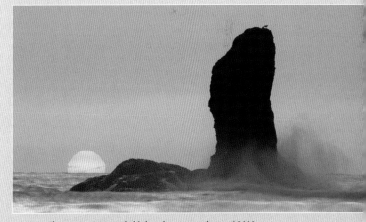

ABOVE: *The ancient Mayans held that the winter solstice of 2012 will bring the end of an era on our planet.*

a universe of numbers

As with any system that provides a way of understanding the world, numerology works within a framework of basic concepts and assumptions which help to give it an internal consistency and a logical basis on which to build, although its most evolved use is intuitional rather than intellectual. Similar concepts are found in a wide range of other disciplines, from physics to psychology, mathematics to religion, but numerology draws them together and works with them in a unique way.

COSMIC VIBRATIONS

One of the underlying principles of numerology is that the universe is filled with energy, and that everything in the universe – whether physical or conceptual – has its own

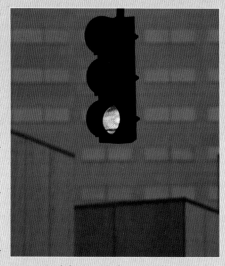

ABOVE: *Symbols are everywhere in our lives. Even the mundane traffic light harnesses the symbolic value of colours to inform and instruct drivers.*

subtle energetic vibrations. Every object has a relationship with every other object by virtue of its particular energy and all resonate with a different vibration. The vibrations in turn create a resonance, or sound, which may or may not be audible to the human ear, and which can be measured scientifically and numerically. The resulting numbers are constants in what appears in many other ways to be an ever-changing world. One of the effects of working with numbers and letters is a

heightened sensitivity to the energy flowing through each number, as it becomes possible to see, feel, or hear this subtle energy.

SYMBOLS

In essence, a symbol is something that represents something else. Usually it is a simple entity – a physical object, a shape, even a colour or number – that is used to signify something complex, conceptual, non-physical or multi-dimensional. For example, the colour red may represent danger, restlessness and fire. In numerology, the numbers are symbols for sets of characteristics, clusters of behaviour, personalities, historical patterns and the relationship between spirit and personality.

Symbols are extremely powerful because they are widely understood and accepted (within a culture or even universally), because they act as a shorthand for something that may otherwise be difficult to understand or express, and because we can often access them both intellectually and at an irrational, subconscious level. In this way they give us many ways to unravel complexity in our lives and to connect with ourselves at a deeper level.

CYCLES

Life has a tendency to show us periods of experience that achieve a stage of completion or fulfilment. Our passage through life is made up of countless cycles, and can itself be seen as a part of the greater cycle of birth, death and rebirth. The nine phases of our lives are made up of three cycles of three nine-year periods – broadly, the birth of the individual, engaging with the world, and engaging with the spirit (which involves introspection and closure). Our time in the womb from conception to birth is a nine-month period which consists of three terms or trimesters. Key developments that occur in the growth of the foetus during each trimester can be seen to parallel the developments that occur through the cycle of numbers.

Our life journey is also mirrored in the constantly changing patterns of nature. Night follows day, and the world sleeps and wakes accordingly. Nature responds to the four seasons in the growth of new life, blossoming, maturing, withering and dying – each year's growth stemming from the growth of previous cycles.

BALANCE AND OPPOSITES

As well as seeing the sequence of numbers one to nine as part of a cycle, we can work with the first eight numbers as odd-even pairs with complementary and contrasting qualities and functions, in much the same way as the Chinese yin-yang

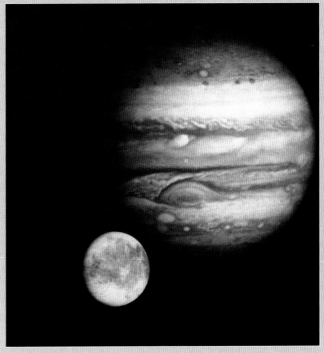

ABOVE: *In astrology, the interaction between the cyclical journeys of the planets around the sun is said to influence our lives.*

symbol shows the interdependence and balance of opposites. Odd numbers possess an active, masculine energy (yang), and work in the realm of the mind and spirit, while even numbers are receptive and feminine (yin), and are associated with earthly, practical matters. The difference between the elements in a pair of such opposites brings into focus both duality and balance.

REDUCTION

One of the most fundamental tools of numerology, reduction, is the simple process of adding the individual digits in a multi-digit number to form a single digit. For example, the number 31 is considered in basic numerological terms to be equivalent to 4; this is arrived at by adding 3 + 1 = 4. In more advanced studies, the reduced number would not be separated from the original, but would be written as 31/4, as this number is different from 13/4, or 22/4. An exception to the rule of reduction is the master numbers – the doubled numbers in the sequence 11, 22, 33... up to 99 – which are sometimes not reduced because of their great potency.

CHAPTER ONE

The Journey
of numbers

Each number from Zero to Nine has significance,
both in itself and as a stage in a cyclical journey.

The numbers build on each other, each gaining resonance and learning from those that have gone before. Nested within the 1–9 cycle are three cycles of three, each containing its own complete journey. The numbers also work as complementary odd-even pairs, though the Nine is unpaired as it provides a culmination and summing up for the previous four pairs. The master numbers 11, 22 and 33 carry a special significance and the appearance of these indicates that one has a special, and perhaps demanding, role to play or task to complete.

When working with numbers, use the interpretations that follow alongside your own perceptions. Be as open as you can, and notice how you feel about the numbers as well as how your feelings change. They will reflect whatever energy you and they are dealing with at the time. Remember that they can be interpreted at more than one level, and the level at which you work at any particular time is the appropriate one for you at that moment. After reading about each number, try to see them all in sequence in your mind's eye, and make a note of any interesting impressions.

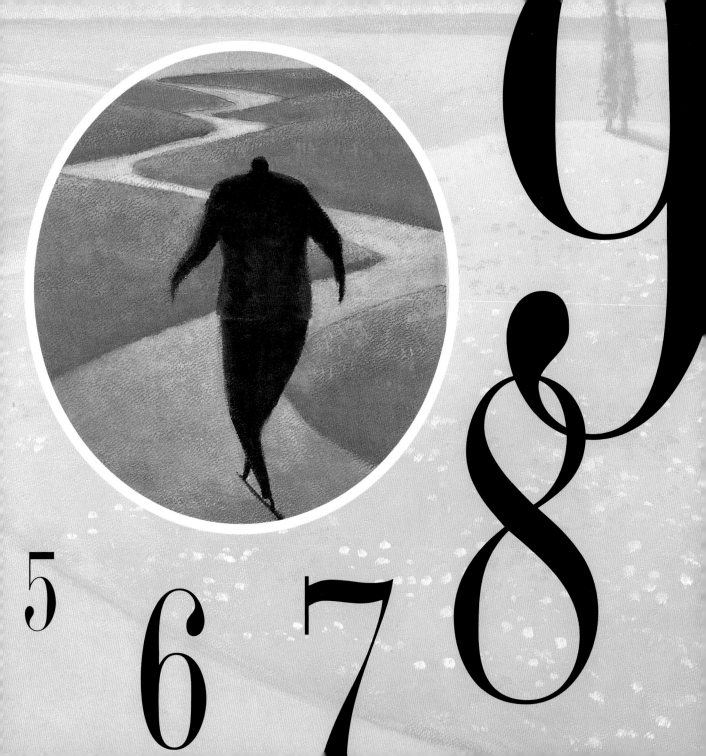

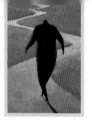

Zero – *the lens*

The all-seeing eye of the Zero observes but does not act, suspended in the hiatus of time and space before the start of a new cycle.

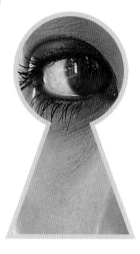

Drawn as a circle, the Zero represents the state before the start of movement and vibration in Number One. We do not work with the Zero in the same way as the other numbers, but it is still important as everything flows from it and eventually returns to it. It contains the memory of all that is past and the possibilities of new creation. It is the juncture at which one cycle ends and the next begins, containing both the closure of the old and anticipation of a new beginning, death and birth or rebirth.

In numerology the Zero is also known as the Lens – it is the all-seeing eye, an entity that sees and

ABOVE: *Like looking through a keyhole, the Zero can see all before him, but cannot react physically to what he sees.*

knows everything that is knowable but cannot act, because it is neither positioned in time and space, nor subject to cause and effect.

Working with this symbol can encourage us to use our reflective faculties. We all have opportunities to enter the Lens from time to time, to withdraw and take stock, before taking our next step in life. The circular form of the Zero tells us that we are faced with both totality and infinite possibility. This happens in particular when we encounter numbers such as 10, 20, or 30. If we were born on the 10th, 20th, or 30th of the month, the ability to withdraw or to go formless may be a regular aspect of our lives, even if we do not use it very much, or very consciously.

LEFT: *The perfect circle of the Zero is called the Lens. Reflecting on the previous cycle and looking forward to the next, it captures the stillness before life and energy burst forth in a new cycle.*

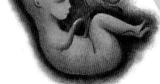

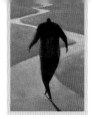

One – *ignition*

At the birth of a new journey or cycle, the pioneering Number One is bursting with ambitious energy.

Number One takes the first step in realizing new possibilities. Each appearance of this number is a rebirth into a new setting or energy environment – it is the flash of a new idea being born, a jet of fire leaving the sun and heading out into the far reaches of space. The pioneering journey of a Number One requires incredible energy, courage and focus of intent as it breaks away from the static state of the Zero.

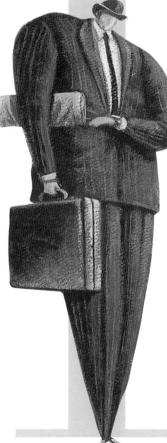

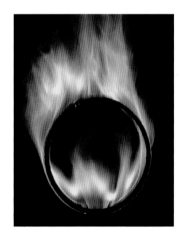

Number One is essentially the principle of action and new growth. It carries the impetus to translate inert potential into something concrete, but it is not the concrete thing itself; it creates possibilities, but leaves the actualization of those possibilities up to others.

Ambitious by nature, a leader in life, the One has an awareness of self as an individual. This awareness, coupled with an innate self-confidence, gives it the inner drive to make its mark, to contribute whatever talents and qualities it may have, even deviant ones. Sometimes it may be living in fear and completely devoid of courage.

FAR LEFT: *Number One is the true original, as it breaks away from the static Zero in a blinding flash of energy and imagination.*
LEFT: *Finding his courage and demonstrating it can provide an example of integrity for others.*

Two − *feeling life*

Relating to the other, the Two tries to balance the emotional seesaw of union and separation.

Number Two represents the next phase of the journey out of the infinite. While there are some things that we may prefer to do alone, perhaps walking in the countryside or sitting in meditation, there are also many other things that require interaction with others. While Number One produces the great new idea, nothing much can be done with it unless others become involved, developing it and giving it form. So we start learning to relate to other people and situations. We begin to experience the world as something outside of ourselves as well as in the deep recesses of our inner selves. In this phase the original sense of unity is lost, and the world can be seen in pairs of opposites: black and white, hot and cold, night and day.

As people try to fulfil themselves through their relationships with others, they encounter a whole range of different experiences as emotions or feelings, ranging from elation to deep depression. Because Number Two is gregarious it can experience separation strongly, and be quick to feel lonely. Indeed it used to be regarded as an unlucky or fateful number specifically because of its association with separation. In its most positive aspect, Number Two is a mediator and seeks to restore unity and peace to the most disparate parts of any situation.

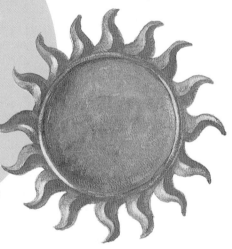

ABOVE AND LEFT:
The Two is constantly aware of duality. Its reward is rediscovering the underlying unity behind everything.

Three — *expressing life*

*Filled with inspiration, the Three expresses
creativity, turning raw feelings into great ideas.*

Number Three represents the completion of the first stage in a tripartite cycle. In the first two phases, there is experience without pattern. But after experiencing life through opposites and extremes, thereby learning the whole gamut of emotions and feelings, it is time to express that great variety of relationships and experiences intellectually as ideas or concepts. Number Three can be flooded by inspiration, but is ultimately lost because it is not grounded. It is an idealistic phase, which is symbolically expressed as a trinity, especially of mother, father and child. The child, resulting from the union of masculine and feminine, represents a potentially higher level of development.

RIGHT: *The Three finds expression
in the archetypal trinity of mother, father
and child. The offspring of the Two's
duality, it offers the potential for even
greater development and expression.*

Number Three translates the raw material of a bright idea, tempered by feeling, into an ideal that has the potential to uplift us all. It is the vital basis of humour, which brings light into the world via the mind. A person who works a lot in Number Three often has an active mind and expresses a wide range of ideas that are frequently clever and witty. Because Number Three produces so many ideas and sees things in unusual or original relationship to each other it can tend to be scattered and lose focus.

IN THE TRIANGLE
*the Three aspires
to a pinnacle of self-
expression from the
stability of its base.*

17

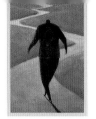

Four — *erecting the structure*

Bringing ideas down to earth is the duty of the Four. With dogged determination, it turns flights of fantasy into reality.

In the third phase we saw a wealth of inspired plans and ideas being expressed powerfully using the creative and intellectual faculties of the mind. We know, though, that turning the original inspiration of a project into tangible reality requires enormous effort. So Number Four is the great number of building and form. It can bring stability and structure but at the same time, because it carries the memory of Number Three, it can hold a vision.

The most important quality needed to bring an idea to fruition is endurance, the ability to overcome obstacles and see things through to completion. This applies not only to practical tasks but also to the journey of the soul that goes through pain and crisis towards a greater understanding of life. Number Four shows great determination to get the job done, but because it tends to be single-minded about its task, conflicts can often occur when working with this number.

The monumental form of the pyramid is associated with this number, drawing inspiration from the heavens through its apex and grounding it in its solid and stable square base.

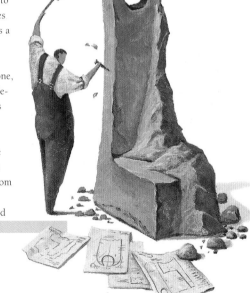

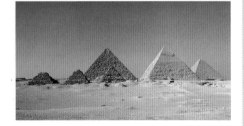

ABOVE: *Four is the builder, turning Three's ideas into something solid and practical.*
LEFT: *The pyramids of Egypt reflect the endurance of the Four, and symbolize its form, giving stability to the Three.*

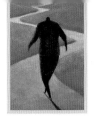
Five — *exploring the structure*

Breaking free from stultifying norms in the quest for knowledge and experience, the Five is on an exciting journey of discovery.

This is the number that occurs midway in our journey from One to Nine. It is the great number of becoming, the movement from what we have built towards the possibility of what we can become.

Number Five works in the element of air and is pre-eminently the number of mind and intellect, pushing back the boundaries of knowledge and communicating this new knowledge to the world. With the frenzy of such important work being done, we can see how the "mad scientist" stereotype could have arisen, through going too deeply and too quickly into the unknown in the pursuit of knowledge.

Five can be restless, impatient for change, wanting to know how things work and how that knowledge might be utilized, but it does not necessarily forget the sense of responsibility so painfully learned in Number Four. The Five's quest for understanding often takes the form of experiencing and evaluating the many facets of life.

It is adaptable and interested in pursuing new perspectives on what is, but not in change for its own sake. It wants to break free from the constraints of what it regards as traditional or conventional life, though it does not necessarily mean that the old values are completely rejected. In fact there is a conflict between the impulse to break free of restriction and the re-booting of the emotional self, which sometimes creates the impression of sentimentality. Faced with such conflicts and with over-whelming choices, the Five can get stuck, and inertia and procrastination can become a problem.

The Number Five is traditionally symbolized by the pentagon. This is the "reliable" square of Number Four unhinged by the addition of another side, creating instability and movement.

NOT CONSTRAINED *by convention, the Five sees new possibilities in existing structures and communicates them with enthusiasm.*

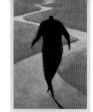

Six – *vision of perfection*

Seeking fulfilment through harmony and perfection, the Six is the idealistic number of heart and home.

The sixth phase marks an important point of culmination and fulfilment at the end of the second cycle of three: things should be as perfect as we can get them. Where Number Five took us on a path that investigates the house that Number Four built, Number Six wants to display the house in a way that reflects its own perfect vision of how it should be. In this phase, the balance of beauty and harmony becomes all-important.

BELOW: *The curly form of the numerically written Six is like a spiral turning in towards its heart.*

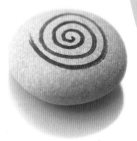

Looking at the shape of the Number Six, we see a curving line spiralling inward to a central point. In this way the number is associated with the heart – either literally the organ at the centre of a human body or the centre of a system such as the Tree of Life. In its association with the family and home, it echoes the mother-father-child trinity of Number Three, the last number in the previous cycle of three.

Number Six encompasses a heady brew of idealism and emotional sensitivity (three twos are six). It can bring to the surface pictures of an idealized world, and with them the potential to uplift us all to a greater vision of who we are. The other side of the coin however, is its obsession and addiction. The beauty of the incoming light can go to our head, and we can mistake the ideal picture of a more beautiful world for reality.

THE STAR OF DAVID *shows the two completed cycles of three superimposed in perfect counterpoint.*

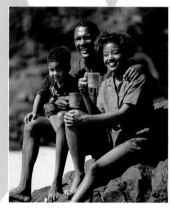

ABOVE: *Domestic harmony and emotional stability are one expression of what motivates the Six.*

20

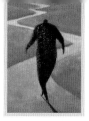

Seven – *realizing perfection*

Mystical transformation can be realized in the spiritual Number Seven, as it seeks to heal life.

Stage Seven of the journey involves translating the Six's ideal vision of the world into something new and tangible. The concept of alchemy – the process of transforming lead into gold in the alchemist's crucible – is useful in understanding the role of the Seven, which involves a spiritual transformation through the mixing and merging of diverse elements and experiences. In this spiritual sense, the changing and deepening of a person's relationship to daily life can result from difficult experiences in the past burning deep into them.

Further pain may be experienced if the transformation is resisted.

Symbolically, Number Seven looks clear in its construction, yet numerically it contains two cycles of three plus a mysterious additional element that gives us the highest and finest expression of those cycles, whether through a deeper understanding of the relationship between the person and the spirit, or through material innovation that can enhance the life of humanity.

Number Seven can make things happen, bringing an element of magic to any situation. Because of the

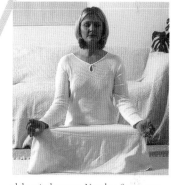

alchemical aspect, Number Seven can be either explosive or moody and experience a profound feeling of being less accomplished than others. Sometimes Number Seven can become absorbed in its own inner world, hence the association with the meditative life and mysticism. Alternatively, it can be obsessed with proving itself and works till it drops.

ABOVE AND LEFT: *The number of spiritual learning, Seven can be introspective and meditative (above), and bring a magical quality to life (left).*

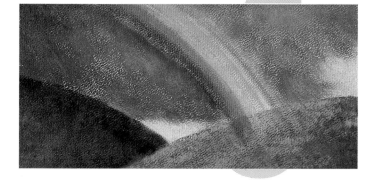

Eight – *perfection reworked*

The strategist and organizer, Eight moves tirelessly back and forth, destroying and rebuilding.

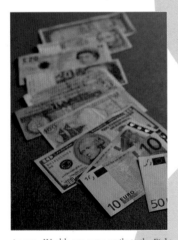

ABOVE: *Wealth can come easily to the Eight.*

In Number Seven we saw how life and spirit combine and mutate to produce the best possible spiritual understanding or material innovation. The role of Number Eight is to find a means whereby everybody can benefit from this – it is a strategist and organizer. It regulates the relationship between spirit and form through its constant movement between the spheres of heaven and earth, cause and effect, time and space, and birth and death. So in the shape of the figure 8 (which, turned on its side, is also the symbol for infinity), energy moves ceaselessly back and forth between two circles. This is a regular movement within a defined space, which gives form to the idea of life moving in cycles or seasons. In a person, this quality can be seen in their tireless energy, spurred on by self-discipline and a competitive spirit.

Number Eight must work in harmony with patterns and with karma (the idea of reaping misunderstandings); if it fails in this it is likely to experience bad luck or even disaster. Like the Four, this number received bad press from many numerologists in the past: people with one or more eights in their birth date were deemed fated to lead generally unfortunate lives. Today we see it in a more positive light: the restriction it brings can be seen as an opportunity to work to uplift that life. Furthermore, this number is strongly associated with regeneration and a good potential for materializing financial wealth through the ability to organize large-scale undertakings.

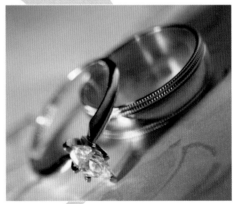

ABOVE: *Two rings, symbols of the eternal commitment of marriage, remind us of the sign of infinity.*

Nine – *the teacher speaks*

Completing the cycle, the Nine achieves fulfilment by dispensing the knowledge of all that has gone before.

Number Nine heralds the completion and fulfilment of the journey of numbers. It carries the whole story of the cycle – all the qualities and characteristics of the numbers that precede it – so in the Nine we look for memory, experience and wisdom.

This number also stands at the threshold of a new journey, poised between endings and beginnings, on the edge of rebirth. It has a quality of transparency as the traveller on this journey must first pass through the Lens of the Zero in Number Ten before a new cycle can begin.

The job of Number Nine is to offer the benefit of its experience and wisdom to those around it. The extent to which this is actually carried out depends on the degree of overall evolution of the soul during the cycle. If the Nine translated its potential wisdom into concrete or intellectual knowledge, it can be difficult for it to move to the silent point of total wisdom and awareness. In order to achieve fulfilment it must learn to move beyond itself: in detachment and self-forgetfulness it remembers all.

LEFT: *In the Nine we find a sense of completion and a transparent quality as it turns its gaze back to the lens of infinite potential.*
RIGHT: *Wisdom gained from experience makes the Nine a truly great teacher.*

the master numbers

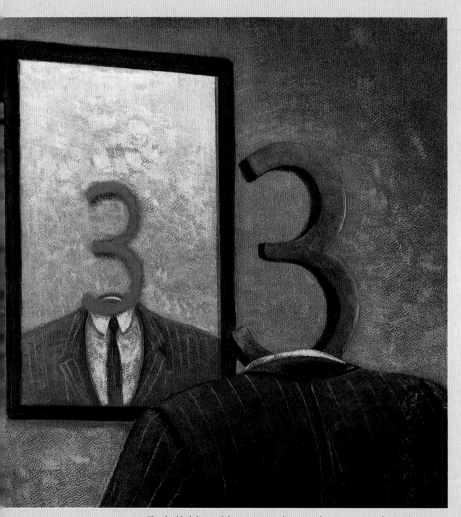

ABOVE: *The doubled digits of the master numbers give them an increased potency.*

Master numbers, or power numbers, are the doubled-digit numbers from 11 to 99. They occupy a special place in numerology as they have a particular power or potency. A master number carries resonances of its two digits as single numbers as well as the number to which it can be reduced. So, for instance, a Twenty-Two has a relationship with both the Two and the Four, and bears characteristics of both. Duplication also gives them a particular potency: as the single digits double themselves they make twice the impact.

The master numbers 11, 22, and 33 embody primary growth or evolution and are often used. The higher master numbers are beyond the scope of this book, largely because they concern refinements of the relationship between the soul and personality.

When derived from a person's name the master numbers are often reduced: the effort of working with the inherited qualities of a master number can be considerable and difficult to sustain, and so using the reduction can make one's life task more manageable. A person's birth, however, can be thought of as an event in the dimensions of time and space, so we work with the particular energies of that moment and tend not to reduce the associated numbers.

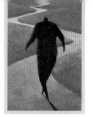
Eleven – *speaking with inspiration*

Deconstructing and reconstructing with intuitive insight, the visionary Eleven accesses the spirit via the most refined aspects of the mind.

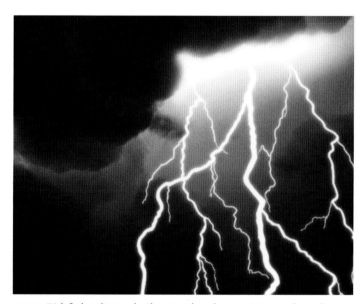

ABOVE: *With flashes of vision, the Eleven translates the raw spirit into understanding.*

the mind. Understanding is elevated to intuition, and spiritual revelation can come as flashes of vision from beyond the rational intellect. This makes Number Eleven seem like a lightning conductor for the spirit, with its clinical intellect able to translate into words a deeper understanding of something that is essentially received in non-verbal form.

When we look at the figure 11, we see two primal symbols of single-pointed, undiluted energy standing in parallel. Expectations are high, and there is no feeling of compromise or vagueness. The job of this number often brings discomfort because it can break up otherwise harmonious patterns of life. Whereas Number Eight does this by destroying and rebuilding in order to regenerate at a higher, but still often material level, Number Eleven takes the ground out from under our feet through the force of intuitive insight, and has been called the number of the prophet at its highest level.

As the first master number or power number, the Eleven has dramatically greater resonance than the numbers in the 1–9 cycle. The Ones contained in the Number Eleven amplify each other, and added together also give it a strong relationship with Number Two. Because of its potency, however, this number is often not reduced.

In practice the Eleven is often involved in learning to channel the spirit via the higher reaches of

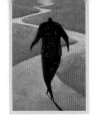

Twenty-two – *building the dream*

From a position of intense sensitivity and fragility, the Twenty-Two can build ever greater and more glorious new structures.

The second master number, Twenty-Two, has a special place both in numerology and in other systems that delve deeper into the meanings and workings of life. There are, for example, 22 major arcana of the Tarot, and 22 paths on the Kabbalistic Tree of Life.

Unlike Number Eleven this master number is often reduced,

BELOW: *The 22 cards of the Tarot's major arcana represent archetypes of humanity.*

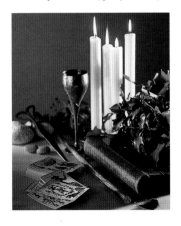

bringing into focus the qualities of Four as well as Two. In the figure 22 the Two looks at its double to see if its creative potential can make something tangible as Number Four. But because of the Two's fragility and sensitivity, this intensity can either bring about a meltdown or cause something new and glorious to arise from it in Number Four. Because of its relationship to Four, Number Twenty-Two is often known as the master builder. If it can keep itself together, then the definite and concrete Four in it can continue to put up newer and greater structures that have solid foundations and embody balance and harmony.

Twenty-Two's qualities are apparent in a person whose quietly systematic approach to life is combined with gentleness and sensitivity.

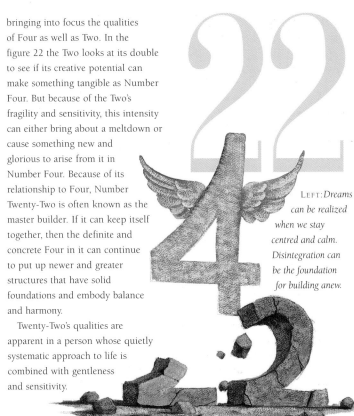

LEFT: *Dreams can be realized when we stay centred and calm. Disintegration can be the foundation for building anew.*

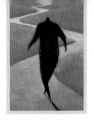

Thirty-three – *ready to give all*

A saint and martyr to good causes, Thirty-Three feels a need to give of itself tirelessly and passionately.

For many people the Thirty-Three can bring great pain or precipitate a crisis as the brilliant light carried by the figure's two Threes illuminates issues of emotional integrity.

This number also contains aspects of the Number Six when reduced, waiting to transform the light of the Thirty-Three into something special, even sacred.

The scope for illusion and the lack of a grip on day-to-day reality in this number are at times considerable. The Six contained in the Thirty-Three is often working in the dark, intermittently receiving from the two Threes a light that lacks shape or direction; because of this, the image of perfection it tries to construct out of this light is illusory. The Thirty-Three's devotion to great causes can become all-consuming, and if a cause proves ultimately unrealizable, despair and hopelessness can quickly set in. At the other end of the spectrum is fanaticism, ultimately a pointless approach to life for which the Thirty-Three runs the risk of earning the label "anti-social".

Not everyone whose numbers include a Thirty-Three will be called to stand on the edge of the abyss of madness. For some the crisis may be a simple question of why they have given such unqualified support to a cause, project or person. A possible answer is that giving something of oneself that could benefit others is sometimes the most appropriate course of action, even in the face of opposition; for this number anything may seem preferable to the emptiness of not giving. When that is understood, the Thirty-Three has realized at least one more point of clarity.

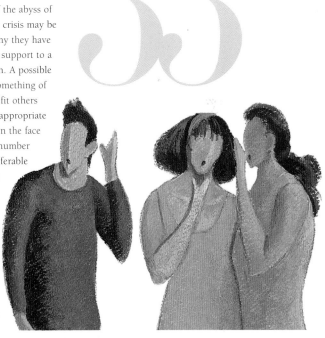

RIGHT: *The passionate conviction of the Thirty-Three can ruffle feathers and lead to ostracism.*

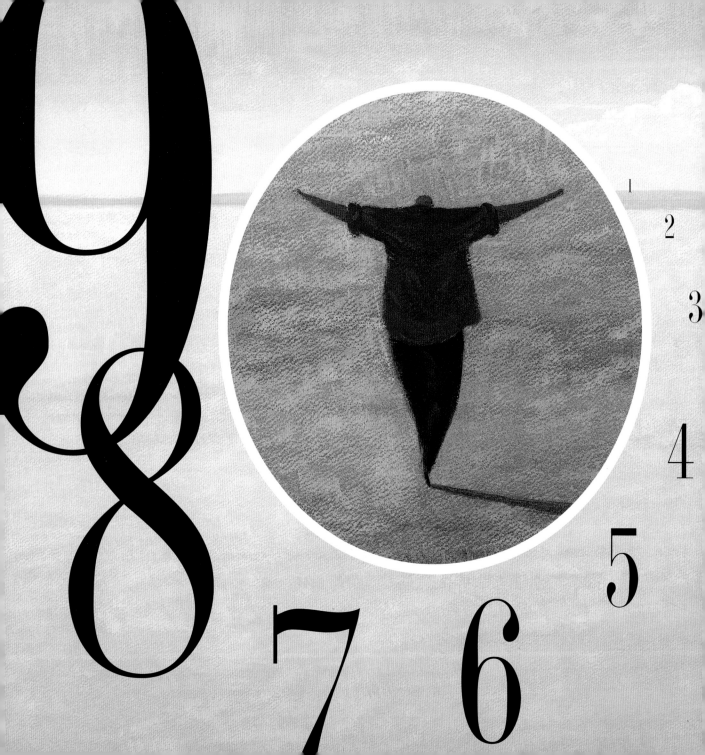

1

2

3

4

5

6

7

CHAPTER TWO

Numbers

in our lives

The numbers found in your name and date of birth can give you fascinating insights into yourself.

Numbers can tell us much about the way we interact with others and with the world, how we approach situations, and how we feel about things.

Our name gives us the Overall Inheritance Number, and this tells us about the traits we inherit from our family and the larger cultural group we were born into. From the day of the month we were born we derive the Evolving Personality Number, which describes the personality traits we have as an individual. The Life Path Number reveals our inner being which drives us in life, and is found by adding all the digits in our birth date. Lastly, the Personal Year Number shows the qualities that are likely to come to the fore in the current year, and is a combination of our birth date and the year of our last birthday.

the overall inheritance number

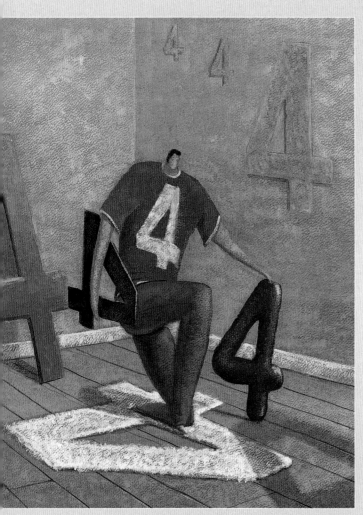

The numerical value of your name represents a blend of spiritual and psychological attributes that you have available in this life and can in many cases be the source of a stereotype. It is determined by your parents, who choose your first names, and by the stories and collective personality of all your predecessors who carried your surname – hence the term Inheritance Number. A child's first name that has already been used in previous generations will serve to reinforce family traits. These days it is common for parents to give their children names that are new in the family or even to invent a name; this can symbolize a break with the past and allow the child to go on its journey less encumbered by family or cultural baggage. By recognizing and using the inherited qualities, the Evolving Personality is better able to do its work, which is to reflect on the aspirations and spiritual energy carried in the Life Path Number and translate them into the reality of a person's life.

To determine the Overall Inheritance Number we generally use the full name that appears on a person's birth certificate. If a person has changed their name, perhaps by marriage or as a result of moving into another culture, or regularly uses a nickname, it is best to look at the values of both the original and the new or alternative names, as the person's life and personality may shift with the change in their identity.

Each letter has a numerical equivalent, as shown below. The value of every letter in the full name should be added together and the final figure reduced to a single digit to determine the Overall Inheritance Number. For example, the name Ann Helen Myers consists of the numbers 1, 5, 5, 8, 5, 3, 5, 5, 4, 7, 5, 9 and 1; these add up to 63, which reduces to 9.

1	2	3	4	5	6	7	8	9
A	B	C	D	E	F	G	H	I
J	K	L	M	N	O	P	Q	R
S	T	U	V	W	X	Y	Z	

30

One – *the leader or loner*

At first glance this number cuts a heroic and courageous figure, not afraid to be outspoken or to stand alone, willing to go where others would not venture. A further look, however, reveals the potential loneliness of a character searching for self-belief and for a certainty of purpose that would enable it to rediscover its heroic role. This is the heritage of this number; its predecessors may well have been leaders in various fields, both intellectual and physical, including areas of work such as medicine. Behind it, though, stands the shadow of self-questioning, of whether its goals can really be achieved.

Two – *the mother hen*

Qualities of nurturing and protection are part of the Two's psyche. The fierce "mother hen" character is often exhibited here – the aspect of Mother Nature that first procreates (by the division of Number One) then protects the children. The inherited experience of pain through separation is carried, but it is also transcended through the need to survive. Life in the water was a physical phase our distant ancestors went through, but we carry the memory of it in the waters of our emotional lives. Living in families, tribes or nations allowed duality to arise and brought about the need to find a central point of balance – hence Number Two's role as mediator. The separation was needed so that a greater diversity of life could be experienced.

Three – *the creative thinker*

In this number feeling seeks expression, but the open side of the figure 3 introduces a degree of vagueness. The shape of the figure resembles two touching semi-circles, or half of the figure 8, hinting at but not realizing the difficulties of the Number Eight. Thus in hereditary terms, the story can be of a stream of creative impulses released in a way that can destabilize families and groups by constantly offering higher but less concrete expressions of creativity.

A tendency to implode and disintegrate matches a continuous planning of new experiments inspired by possibility. There is a serendipity about the number, an innocence which makes opposite sides of the same coin equally possible and equally appealing.

The Three is always trying out new ways of doing things and of perpetuating possibility, rather than choosing a path and sticking with it. Many Threes will come with inheritances in the creative arts, which lift thought above material form and back towards the original inspiration.

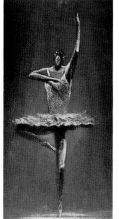

LEFT: *Creative arts are often part of the Three's background, giving it an essential outlet for self-expression.*

Four – *the worker*

The shape of the figure 4 shows two sides of a triangle extending outward. This gives a feeling of stability as it suggests that the creative potential of Number Three has been anchored or rooted and cannot easily fly away. The Number Four's discipline and determination to get the job done can mean that it rides roughshod over others in the process, and this has created an inheritance which sometimes carries stories of conflict within and between families and groups. Looked at positively, such conflict can serve to break up the inherited patterns of behaviour or disease that characterize a family, for example, bone and joint problems that can be associated with rigid thought patterns. The feuds that are sometimes carried on over generations will in time find resolution; this brings greater compassion in its wake and the karmic rhythm of life is then better understood.

Five – *the restless intellectual*

The shape of the figure 5 evokes the feeling of movement. Usually this is not random movement but motion with a purpose, unless it is in a flat spin. Five is the number that explores and moves us out of the rigidity of Number Four. The inheritance of those carrying this number may tell of ancestors who travelled extensively, in some cases opening up previously unknown parts of the world. The Five is also sometimes associated with the scribe, the keeper of the records of families, groups, countries and civilizations. It can bring a wide-ranging intellect to bear upon a variety of questions, and draws on the breadth of experience that it seeks out.

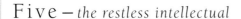

RIGHT: *Movement and frantic intellectual activity characterize the Number Five.*

Six – *loyalist or traitor*

Number Six identifies with the story of how families with a strong bond subsequently split up, leaving a legacy of insecurity. Loyalty and betrayal often feature large, the latter being the quality that provokes change. However, betrayal can become a habit that permeates a family through many generations.

In time, though, six focuses its attention on refining thought and sensibility, and developing a more elevated view of how the world could be. This is the quest for perfection, as an ideal of family life.

The Six's emotional harmony may be disrupted by the protective aspect of this number, which can breed jealousy. The gift, though, is the uplifting of life through the heightening of our sense of beauty.

Seven – *the abstract thinker*

Seven's developed intellect stabilizes the emotional sensitivity that is felt inside, and this sometimes makes it seem cold and aloof. Explosiveness and unexpressed bitterness can become issues both in family and in larger groups, but as the Seven's material world slowly expands and reason emerges, the bitterness can be dissolved. This number gains wisdom from the past and a capacity for abstract thought. It realizes that universal energy is experienced through events, and how you cope with a particular event or person is really how you respond to the associated energy.

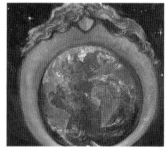

ABOVE: *Cosmic affairs interest the Seven.*

Eight – *the transformer*

The inheritance of this number brings the destruction of old, restrictive ways of life and the generation of new patterns. Eight has often been associated with bad luck, seemingly the victim of events outside its control, but in fact these apparently external forces are a reflection of its internal world. For example, patterns of ill health experienced by successive generations in a family or ethnic group may seem to result from a genetic predisposition but actually arise from bad habits that cause "disease" to be passed on. The patterns can be repeated for all eternity and the resulting affliction accepted as fate, or they can be challenged, reworked in a more harmonious, spiritual way, and overcome. Inherited misunderstandings about the relationship between the spirit and physical life can thus be dissolved.

With its heritage of strong intellect, organization and control over financial matters, Number Eight may well have a legacy of large business enterprises and wealth, developed and passed down through generations.

RIGHT: *At ease in big business, the Eight is traditionally associated with wealth and materialism.*

Nine – *the sage*

Because of the Nine's broad spectrum of characteristics, many of the stories of the preceding numbers can apply to varying degrees here. Beyond that, its job may be concerned with showing how the past has been digested and understood. Nines have played important roles as historians and philosophers, either in the formal academic sense or in assumed roles within a family, community or nation. Number Nine can be characterized as the wise man or woman, though in some cases wisdom and experience can be overlaid with cynicism or affected naïvety. This is natural, particularly as memory turns into understanding, but it can also be used as a deliberate technique to avoid looking at an issue straight on.

Eleven — *the inspired warrior*

For much of the time, the person with the Eleven emerging from their name may well be working with its reduced counterpart, Number Two, because the demands of this master number are so great. The Eleven can bear the burden of responsibility for difficult changes within a family group over time, which may be reflected through alterations to the genetic code itself. This is achieved through being open to a higher vision, reflected in both material and intellectual advances over time, and carrying through this vision. The Eleven will often have encountered resistance because the changes involved didn't always seem logical at first, even if they were later seen as inspired.

Twenty-Two — *the master builder*

The relationship between Number Twenty-Two and its reduced version, Number Four, is not straightforward. The Number Two that looks at itself can tend towards thoughtfulness, even introspection, and reveal little of the fruits of its deliberations. In terms of inheritance, it can bring the quality of elegant and deeply felt work to the fore. The inheritance can demonstrate what was done to raise the effort of everyday life to as high a level as possible. Within the family group, the number can show how vision and skill can be combined with endurance to produce something that uplifts. If the number becomes introverted, stasis, disconnection and conflict can result.

BELOW: *The Twenty-Two shares some of the Two's concerns with duality and opposites.*

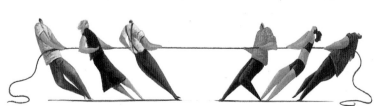

Thirty-Three — *the helper*

The "unappreciated artist" syndrome can arise here, but this is more to do with how the person with this number in their inheritance feels about themselves than any strict definition of what constitutes art. It could apply equally to the manager of a supermarket as to a stereotypical figure in a garret working with oils and canvas.

As an inheritance it can encourage a family or other group to raise its aspirations and understand that it is better to "reach for the stars" and fail than not to try at all. However, irrespective of the views of others and of its own achievements, the Thirty-Three will often have a tendency to judge itself a failure because it knows that there is an even greater picture to be painted, and its reduction, the Six, says that the painting could be more beautiful.

the evolving personality *number*

You can learn more about your personality from the day of the month you were born. The difference between this number and the Overall Inheritance Number lies in the origins of the characteristics. The Inheritance Number originates in your social context (family, tribe etc), while the Evolving Personality Number is more forward-looking, and recognizes that with the passing of time the personality is learning, becoming refined and developing. It is the outward expression of your inner being, your interface with the external world, and is influenced by your journey through life.

With this number, pinpointing your key traits – well-balanced, self-centred, idealistic, practical and so on – becomes easy. But while the basic traits will stay with you throughout your life, the Evolving Personality Number does allow you the flexibility to change and grow. Knowing where you are starting from and the direction you are moving in helps the evolution of the personality. For instance, if you are approaching a point of crisis because you have opened yourself to spiritual growth, you will more easily understand that your personality needs to become more inwardly directed to cope with the difficulties of change.

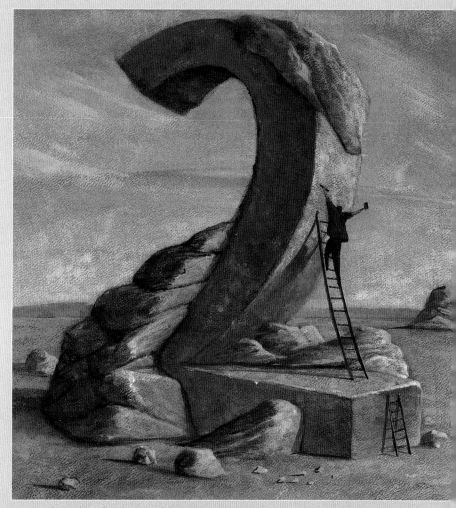

ABOVE: *The numbers of our birth date help us discover and express core personal qualities.*

One — *birth dates: 1st, 10th, 19th and 28th*

One brings a burning drive to make its mark on life, to display its strong sense of self and individuality. It can be important to distinguish self-absorption from selfishness; this preoccupation with the self can result in loneliness or attention-seeking. The focus on the individual may appear as reluctance to stand alone, and with that, passivity, procrastination and an unwillingness to develop a real sense of self. In relationships, difficulties can arise when a Number One has a strong will to drive an idea through to acceptance. Wit, straight-talking and brash assertiveness may be smoke-screens for insecurity.

A One may respond to early challenges by rebelling or with-drawing. Later, its need to test and prove itself often creates a pattern of seeking out fresh challenges; however, if it feels that it will fail to meet a challenge it is likely to delay and make excuses.

As an evolving vibration, Number One increasingly shows innovation and independence, possessed by a drive to act for the collective good rather than the self.

Key traits: individuality, independence, wilfulness, self-centredness.

ONE has a burning drive to make an impression.

Two — *birth dates: 2nd, 20th and 29th*

Those born under the influence of this number are emotionally sensitive. Their development involves learning to understand the virtues of this sensitivity, and not simply experiencing it as pain from which bitterness can develop. They can allow themselves to feel crushed, and wear their vulnerability like a badge.

The same sensitivity can be used to appreciate different points of view and to help bring people together. This quality enables the Two to act as mediator or diplomat, and to hold together all the diverse elements of a situation, though it may achieve its aims through being manipulative if it cannot do so through gentle persuasion. The Two "feels" things out and tries to make sense of them. If the process is painful, it may take things personally. Its sensitivity to duality can also make it indecisive.

Key traits: sensitivity, vulnerability, diplomacy, manipulation.

ABOVE: *The yin-yang symbolizes the Two's balancing and mediation of opposites.*

Three — *birth dates: 3rd, 12th, 21st and 30th*

Those carrying the Number Three vibration can feel a restless creativity striving to be expressed. They can also seem moody: having taken on board the feelings experienced by Number Two, the Three expresses the full spectrum, from elation to despondency. This number's job is to remould and crystallize these feelings creatively through an illuminated intellect: feelings must be given shape and articulated. From the Three's urge to rise and fly there sometimes emerges a refined intellect with piercing insight, and a cleverness which can be deployed so as to hide hurt feelings. This intellectual capacity can be turned to exaggeration and elaborate, entertaining story-telling. The Three's exuberance is expressed in extravagance and luxury, affection and generosity.

Key traits: creativity, insight, intellect, wit, moodiness.

Four — *birth dates: 4th, 13th and 31st*

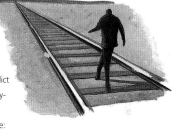

The personality that develops within this vibration works with perseverance and an ability to hold things together. The visions of the Threes are anchored in a usable form. Good organizers, Number Fours prize reliability and will work long and hard to translate the vision into a lasting form or structure. Because this work requires perseverance, some Fours can be seen as rigid and unwilling to compromise. As a result conflict often arises from within this vibration, originating in anything from slight awkwardness to downright bloody-mindedness on the part of the Four. Resistance to change can lead to this number getting into a rut.

Hard work, frugality, routine and orderliness are important to Fours. This conservatism can be a hindrance: sometimes they have difficulty accepting others whose values, standards or methods are different, so are hard taskmasters. As they are reluctant to take risks they can miss out on opportunities – and regret it.

Key traits: perseverance, practicality, rigidity, resistance to change.

ABOVE: *Fours have staying power on long and complex projects.*

Five — *birth dates: 5th, 14th and 23rd*

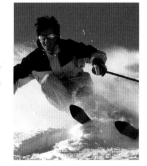

Often an individualist who will not be pinned down, the Five deals with issues of experience. The Five works with unusual ideas and concepts, even sexual promiscuity. Fives seek excitement and novelty, and get along well with everyone, making them attractive to others. However, they do not hang around for long, and may move on in haste for fear of becoming too attached.

Number Five is a persuasive communicator, but the value of its communications can be suspect. For instance, a politician may seem earnest about believing in a cause, but his words are basically a means to a different end, not a literal expression of belief. So in this role the Number Five should aim to develop the qualities of accountability and integrity.

In keeping with their restless energy and their strong communication skills, Fives can often be found in careers involving travel, sales, performing sports and science.

Key traits: freedom, individuality, communication.

ABOVE: *Excitement and novelty are the food and drink of the Five.*

Six — *birth dates: 6th, 15th and 24th*

The Six's intense experience of life can bring anxiety and low self-esteem. Its association with the family makes empathy and consideration natural traits, but it needs to learn balance before it will find happiness here. Sixes are often found in the caring professions or working in the service of others; in their personal lives, altruism taken to excess may result in them interfering in other people's lives, or being used. They are loyal and supportive, and protection of standards is important to them. The evolution of the personality comes as their vision grows larger and less personal.

Key traits: intensity of experience, empathy, loyalty, self-negativity.

Seven — *birth dates: 7th, 16th and 25th*

This number combines extreme fragility with an ability to make things happen. The Seven constantly seeks to balance two apparently contrasting aspects: a deeply private inner world and a restless drive to materialize things innovatively. Inner loneliness and intense reflection result from the struggle to render the inner and outer life as one. A periodically deep sense of inadequacy is compensated for by furious activity. With a well-developed intellect, this number forms opinions on the basis of observation and reason rather than emotion. The Seven is also at ease with the world of mystery and spirituality, but tends to approach it in a scientific way and when frustrated may turn sceptic. Sevens

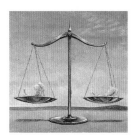

steer clear of frivolity and superficiality, preferring a more in-depth approach to life and people; they may, however, miss out on the joys of life if they are too single-minded in this approach. They can have a marked talent for innovation and invention.
Key traits: fragility, internal conflict, love of nature, intellect, emotional aloofness.

LEFT: *Seven balances inner and outer life.*

Eight — *birth dates: 8th, 17th and 26th*

Working with this vibration can generate conflict because the Eight forces reassessment of its surroundings and is eventually compelled to reassess itself. Conflict stems from resistance to change or from forcing change and provoking resistance in others. Number Eight is a powerful figure that can build, destroy and build anew to improved specifications. It has vision and a strong will, and can see things on a grand scale; can take on the role of leader, especially in business. Its ability to understand intuitively what motivates others helps it in this role, though it can also channel this ability to self-interest. Number Eight can be conservative and opinionated, and may appear prickly or pushy, even ruthless.
Key traits: leadership, discipline, conflict, pushiness.

Nine — *birth dates: 9th, 18th and 27th*

All the qualities of the preceding numbers are contained in the Nine, so it combines strong emotions with clear thinking. It is inspirational, inclined to paint life on a large canvas and not to get bogged down in small day-to-day details. As the last number in the cycle, the Nine can experience an urgent need for fulfilment mingled with a pervasive feeling of emptiness, which signals the proximity of the Lens and the return of the Number One in a new cycle.

As they develop a sense of perspective, people in this vibration stand back a little to get an overview of a situation before acting. Number Nine looks forward to the next cycle and this lends it an air of optimism and dreamy idealism.

This number can vacillate between naïvety and cynicism in like measure, until it remembers that both qualities are part of the same story to which it has contributed. Then it stands between the two at a point of steadiness, from where it can respond to others with openness and generosity.
Key traits: strong emotions, idealism, clarity, feelings of emptiness, naïvety, cynicism.

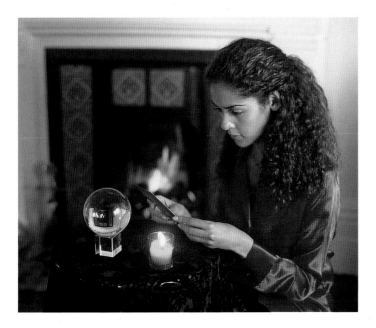

Twenty-Two —
birth date: 22nd of the month

The relationship between earth and water can be a challenge here because we look at Number Twenty-Two both as it stands and as the reduced Number Four. The internal dialogue between the two Twos means that the deep waters of the emotions are felt but may not be expressed, because an appropriate language does not seem to exist.

Better therefore, to lose oneself in the hard work of building life through Number Four, whether in business, the professions or the arts.

This vibration can bring a compassionate insight to organizations and institutions because the Number Twenty-Two functions primarily through feeling. It can also bring nervous breakdown, though the Number Four will tend to use the sensitive energy to put down firm psychological or physical foundations.
Key traits: hard work, compassion, inability to express emotions.

ABOVE LEFT: *The Eleven gains insight through intuition.*

Eleven — *birth dates: 11th and 29th of the month*

For those born on the 11th, there is often an issue of how intellectual process and feeling relate. It deals with primordial force roaring through it. The pure Eleven needs to stand its ground and not be moved by mere reason, as within its perspective there is a greater view of the world than that dictated by logic. That greater view can be realized through the awakening intuition. Others may experience the pronouncements of the insightful Eleven as stubbornness, and indeed sometimes the Eleven may have to defer, accepting that the world is not yet ready for its new insight. They are a vehicle of revelation, but not the revelation itself. Cynicism and the emergence of occult knowledge can cast a long shadow. The Eleven may have to remember that, in time, everything finds its right place in the order of things.
Key traits: intuition, insight, cynicism.

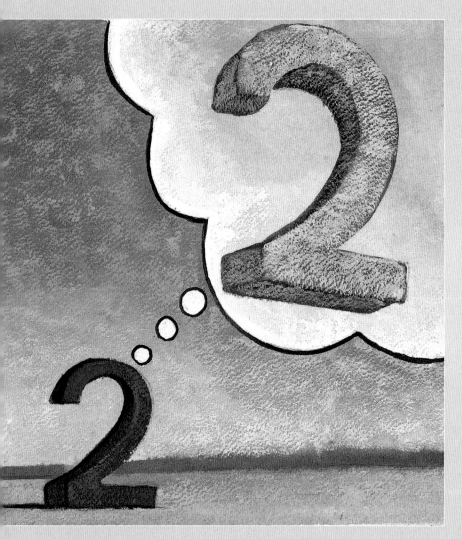

The Life Path Number is the most important number in a numerology chart. It symbolizes the aspiration of the soul to express in the world its highest, most spiritual qualities, which it does through the medium of the evolving personality. In the Life Path Number lies your latent potential, and an awareness beyond everyday mundane issues. Whereas the Evolving Personality Number can be seen as your outer nature, or how you present yourself in the world, this number represents your private, inner self, your intrinsic, essential qualities.

You may feel this as a yearning to develop in a particular way, and you may also resonate with this number when you feel that you are achieving your purpose in life.

This number is obtained by adding up all the numbers in your date of birth – for example the birth date 29th July 1969 is added and reduced as follows: $(2 + 9) + (7) + (1 + 9 + 6 + 9) = 43$; 43 reduces to 7, so the Life Path Number in this example is 43/7. $2 + 1 + 1 + 9 + 7 + 3$

02 01 1973 $= 23/5$

$= 5$

LEFT: *The life path number reveals the higher, spiritual qualities which our souls yearn to express.*

One – *the selfless will to act*

In Number One as a Life Path Number, the will to act is entirely selfless, and only slowly and by degrees will this great, dispassionate, fiery urge to create be recognized, integrated, and put to use by the evolving personality. This aspect of the number can precipitate an existential crisis as it faces the dilemma of whether to develop an independence of spirit and a strong will for the self, family and community, or to hand over the reigns and allow the spirit to manifest through the self as it will.

Two – *duality*
seeking unity

The highest spiritual aspect of the number is the part that is in contact with the divine, and Number Two has an innate tendency to search for God and a unity with God. It knows that there is a purpose behind the descent into the forgetfulness of materialism: it needs to learn through experience that a deeper understanding of oneness or unity is achieved through the illusion of thinking that this oneness is lost.

The spiritual aspect of Number Two experiences the duality of gender but seeks to rediscover the unity of the point of no gender – a position which was held in Number One, and the possibility of which we saw in the Lens. Something of this can be seen in practice, for instance, when a woman shows masculine qualities such as assertiveness, or a man finds his feminine/receptive aspect. Here the Two finds a balance of opposites, which is an alternative way of addressing duality.

Three – *a greater*
conception of life

Number Three in its highest aspect is about the birth of a greater conception of life than in previous numbers. In the moment of conception, oneness is revisited. The child is the fruit of that moment, containing a balance of both masculine and feminine aspects, and symbolizes hope for a better world. The idealized notion of the Trinity of mother, father and child carries a natural stability resulting from the union of the two genders, rather than the instability found in the notion of "three's a crowd". From within this framework of stability the Three can safely work with its creative energy, including its sexuality. If it is inhibited in its attempts to do so, it may destroy or abandon its own creations, or channel its energies into building up a false sense of stability in its material surroundings.

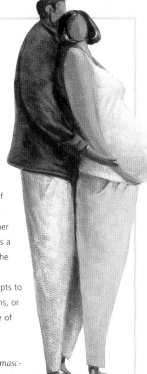

RIGHT: *The child is the fruit of the union between masculine and feminine, and has the potential for greater things.*

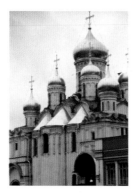

Four – *carrying the light of the spirit in material form*

In the Life Path Number, the Number Four has the ability to realize its creative aspect through the evolving personality. The Four's quest is to transform the spirit into its day-to-day physical form. At its highest level, Number Four expresses itself through intuition, but the fruits of this intuition must be grounded in daily life for the Four to be satisfied. As our planet Earth harbours the light and heat of the sun, so Number Four carries the light of the spirit in the material form, goes through the resultant burning, and declares the material life blessed. Some of the great cathedrals and temples on the planet attempt to do just that. The creative arts and related activities are a fertile field for those working in this vibration, but the creativity associated with the Number Four occurs within a well-defined framework, rather than as abstract expression.

LEFT: *The builder, Four, creates great monuments to spirituality, giving it physical expression.*

Five – *at the gateway to humanity's divine nature*

Number Five in its greatest aspect is the gateway to humanity's divine nature. It is the mind of God coming into the human mind. There has always been a dream that we could be something greater than we are now, transcending the physical and psychological laws that we have accepted as truth. If Five is a number strongly associated with the senses, then its lesson is to transcend sensuality, to find a balance between this and the Four's constrictions, between body and soul. This can also mean learning to recognize when the time is right to move on to a new experience and when to stay and learn more from the current situation.

Most of us are familiar with the legend of Superman and with other fictional heroes who appear in cultures around the world. They are unusually benign beings who work for the good of the many rather than for personal gain; thus they symbolize both freedom from karmic restriction and the selfless quality of the evolved Number Five.

Six – *spiritual harmony*

The great Number Six takes the light of higher understanding and translates it as pure wisdom. The obsessional, addictive aspects of the number, which can precipitate crisis at the evolving personality level, are released by stages. Eventually we are liberated from the physical senses, and the only addiction to remain is intoxication with the ideal of God.

This number is traditionally associated with marriage, home and family. In the Life Path Number, this manifests itself as the symbolic union of the active, spiritual principle with the creative, receptive principle, of the spirit and the personality. The two triangles of the six-pointed Star of David symbolize this balance and union. We find our own heart centre and heartbeat, and know that all aspects of life can come together at this point.

Seven – *spiritual understanding*

The deep understanding of what happens when material life merges with the pure spiritual fire, when the rational mind and the intuitive heart become integrated, is the prize offered by this number. It represents the end of the association with nature at a physical level in the cycle, and the development of self-awareness that nature itself does not have – beyond this, the numbers are concerned with the intellect and the spirit. Introspective and meditative, the Seven tries to understand the changing make-up of its being, but true insight is just beyond reach as there is always another layer waiting to be revealed. The association of this number with mysticism and the priesthood comes from the internal alchemical work that it does. Spiritual transformation may be a painful process, as all the elements must be combined and heated before emerging on another level of awareness.

Eight–
to rule is to serve

The Eight takes what it is given and reprocesses or transforms it into regular patterns of energy. Right in the centre of the Eight, at the crossover, is the point of transformation, of death and regeneration, which we pass through and which offers the possibility of spiritual refinement and heightened awareness. In time, the Eight's feeling of being in servitude to the cycle of life and death gives way to the higher knowledge that we can guide others in navigating the variable waters of life. In short, it learns to wield power wisely and for the benefit of all.

Nine – *processing the memory of life*

This number is both the end of one road and the beginning of a new one. Even as it draws in and rolls up the experiences and understanding of a whole cycle, the Nine is becoming increasingly transparent, making for the rebirth of fire in Number One. It has to learn to let go of things willingly, and for the Nine more than any other number, it is important to realize that life is depersonalized. The weight of memory can become a burden, but a person can deal with it by consciously being part of the universal Number Nine, containing and processing the memory of the whole of life carried in the solar system and beyond. With this comes the ability to be the true humanitarian and help everyone realize their full spiritual potential.

RIGHT: *Letting go is one of the most important lessons for the Nine, otherwise memories become a burden.*

Eleven – *the prophet*

This number has atomized the past but knows that those same atoms carry the knowledge and experience of the preceding cycle. In its highest understanding Number Eleven carries mystery in the space between its two Ones, which is bordered with fire, creating potential for a new cycle of time to commence.

The relationship between the past that has been worked through and expressed, on the one hand, and its new position in a fresh matrix of time and space, on the other, gives rise to the vision of the prophet. This vision describes the characteristics of the new cycle as it lies dormant; the prophet sees its qualities reflected in the light of the fire and declaims them.

The flame of Number Eleven identifies with a view of the past, and with the possibilities of how the genetic code might develop in the future. All those possibilities are seen in this number before the measuring of life through time restarts.

ABOVE: *The fiery conductor rods of Eleven transmutes the potential for a new cycle to start moving.*

Twenty-Two – *the master builder*

In its greatest understanding, this number shows us that feelings of separation and loss really are an illusion. By constantly looking at itself, this number's doubled digits cannot forget that they were born out of love and unity. For the Two, simply looking at its own reflection is not enough, however; the Twenty-Two must give rise to something concrete, and this is how it relates to the Number Four which is reduced from it. At this level, the Twenty-Two is about building greater awareness in humanity in its material environment, and for this reason the Number Four – planet Earth if you like – needs to be transformed. As our understanding of ourselves and our universe deepens and broadens, the edifice of enlightenment and understanding is built higher through us. Through the way we live our lives, we all contribute to the work of this number.

Thirty-Three – *the true sacrifice*

It is sometimes said that the greatest sacrifice lies in giving up those beliefs and values that we hold most dear. In other words, if we can progressively release the illusions that bind us to this world, then the Number Six that reduces from Thirty-Three becomes the carrier of unconditional wisdom and understanding. We can feel ourselves alternately burdened by a heavy material world, and lost in abstractions

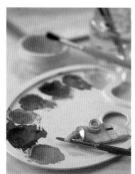

of that world. It may seem a noble aspiration to see life as art, but we must also remember that art moves in fashions. If it is true that life cannot ultimately be experienced as art at all, that it can be expressed only as wisdom through intuition, then the sacrifice is indeed terrible. In its highest expression, however, the Thirty-Three works for a truer understanding of the divine within us all.

LEFT: *Life as art is a common aspiration, but one that is ultimately illusory.*

the personal year number

0+2 + 01+2011 ~ 7

Unlike the Overall Inheritance, Evolving Personality and Life Path numbers, this number has significance for a period of a year only. Derived from the day and month of your birth plus the year of your most recent birthday, the Personal Year Number is applicable from birthday to birthday.

This number reveals the potential for what can happen during the year. Work with it constructively and you could achieve your goals more fully, or avoid the frustration of running up against a brick wall. You can use it to choose the best time to do things or to make major changes in your life, for example looking for a new job, moving house or starting a relationship. Conversely it can also be a useful indicator of when to hold tight and delay making a major change. You can also use it in a more general sense to help you focus on particular personal issues such as health, relationships with others, or your material well-being.

As the Personal Year Number repeats in nine-year cycles, each number will come up several times for you, and each time it will provide particular learning opportunities within the context of your ever-changing life. You will need to grasp these opportunities if you are to break out of patterns and avoid repeating the same lessons each cycle.

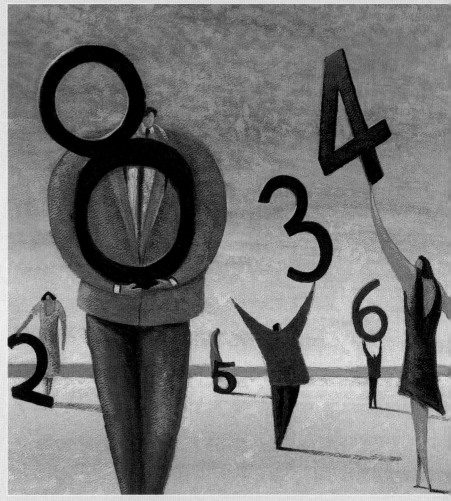

ABOVE: *The personal year number helps us all to work in harmony with unfolding events.*

One – *fresh beginnings*

This year is filled with opportunities, burning and purifying the memories of the preceding cycle. Wipe the slate clean and start anew, converting dreams and ideas into reality; now could be a good time to change career or move house. During this year it is important to act decisively, avoiding hesitation and procrastination. To do this you may need to address old fears or habits that prevent you from getting things done. Health-wise, look out for the wellbeing of the spine and back together with circulation below the knee, as problems in these areas can impede the forward march of the spiritual warrior. Emotionally it is a good time to start new relationships and clarify existing ones, either by strengthening and deepening them or by jettisoning them if they are holding you back.

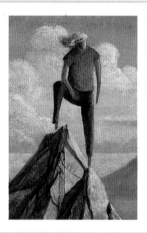

RIGHT: *The progress of the spiritual warrior can be impeded by physical problems or stale relationships.*

Two – *finding peace*

The year ahead can usefully be focused on nurturing the ideas and activities that were brought into focus or fruition in the previous year, and finding peace within yourself and with others.

Confusion and psychic disturbance may result from your energy being pulled in different directions, and from the appearance of choices needing to be made. The key is to go for unifying factors – when there seem to be several options or alternatives, step back and look at the bigger picture, the underlying unity behind what you encounter. Consider whether taking sides is helpful, and be the peacemaker and conciliator. See how the feminine qualities of life can be exalted: uplift others with empathy, and refrain from force. With the emotions to the fore, this is a good time for relationships. But psychic perception can be accentuated and caution may be needed in its use.

Three – *self expression*

The year should be one of creativity, fun and expansive goodwill. It is time to crystallize ideas that come from a point of inspiration, so beware of the tendency to scatter your energies in too many different directions. While this is a social number, and the year should bring joy through contact with others, keep a focus in your relationships.

In a Number Three Personal Year you can uplift others into their higher, spiritual selves, and at the same time let them rediscover themselves. In life, you should go for the creative potential of your life that really moves you, and focus on self-expression.

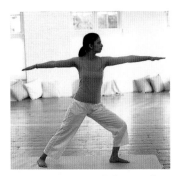

ABOVE: *In a Four year find peace within.*

Five – *exploring new possibilities*

This is an auspicious time for making changes, exploring different ideas, meeting new friends, perhaps trying a new relationship; bear in mind, though, that during this period it may be difficult to stay faithful. Business endeavours can prove financially rewarding. If you do take risks on the business front, watch out for tendencies to be either impulsive or indecisive – with a richness of possibilities to explore, choices can become overwhelming and procrastination may paralyse. There is however, a chance both to get and to give a perspective on the world beyond the confines of your usual daily life. Number Five enables you to speak (or write) your mind more freely, and the more that it carries the imprint of your own truth, the greater its impact will be.

Four – *discipline and consolidation*

This is not a time for launching new initiatives or for spreading largesse to the world at large. Rather consolidate what you have, tidy things up, put your affairs in order, and keep on top of the job. When hostility or opposition comes your way, let forbearance and endurance be your watchwords. This is also a year for disciplined creativity. If, for example, you are a composer, be mindful of form and structure, respecting your musical roots – leave experimentation for another year! Look for your peaceful centre inside, perhaps through meditation, in order to counter the stress that can arise from working too hard.

Six – *winds of change*

The Six brings change: relationships may end, but equally the time could be ripe for marriage or other long-term commitments. During this cycle, the integrity of the family unit (or similar group) can thus be a sensitive issue, and may take priority over personal needs. Which way things go will depend on how the number functions. Its

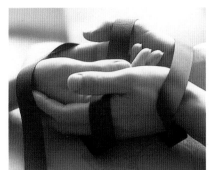

natural course is to aim for the "marriage" in the centre and a deepening of the relationship, but if understanding doesn't match feeling, there can be fracture or "divorce".

LEFT: *Changes to the status quo could mean a deepening and formalizing of relationships – or a split if feelings are not fully understood.*

Seven — *soul-searching*

This is a time to be aware of the potential for illusion. It is also a good time to see a project through to a satisfactory conclusion because this number has the unique capacity to blend external and internal factors. Frustration and the appearance of darkness can make life seem grim, but it is only your subconscious mind saying, "explore this power and use it". Feelings can well up and subside quickly; let this happen and learn from it. You do not need to wear your vulnerability on your sleeve. This is a good time for both material or financial wellbeing and soul-searching; part of the magic of the Seven is that both are possible. With all your preoccupations, there can be misunderstandings in relationships during this phase, and you will need to make sure you have time to yourself.

BELOW: *In the Seven year soul-searching and the pursuit of material comfort are not mutually exclusive.*

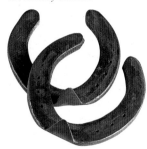

Eight — *going with the flow*

This is a phase over which you cannot exercise much control, so take what life throws at you, be it good luck or bad, and work with it constructively in the knowledge that it is an expression of the universe readjusting itself and moving up a gear.

The year is marked by money and power, so even if you need to shrug off some unexpected setbacks, it is a good time for business and money-making plans to take off, and you could well win at gambling.

Ill-health and stress may arise in relationships, either in your own life or in the life of someone you know well. Don't get frustrated; practise detachment and get to know the still point at the centre of your being. Walk the middle path between infinity and daily life, aware of both, but owned by neither.

ABOVE: *Good and bad luck may come your way in an Eight year. Either way you will need to work with them.*

Nine — *resolution*

The third cycle of three is now done, so now is the time to let understanding filter through as you draw together the strands of what has gone before. Try to resolve any unresolved issues, for example at home or in the workplace. Clear the decks for a new start. If there have been incidents that left you hurt or angry, and that still bother you, come to peace with them now. It is also a time for forgiving and letting go, in preparation for a new cycle. In this period, others may come seeking your help with their problems; in a Number Nine energy, you can afford to give them the benefit of your experience.

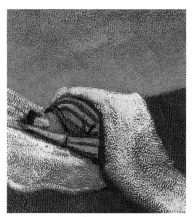

Eleven — *intuition and dynamic meditation*

You can afford to stand your ground in this period, in the knowledge that through this number you may be perceiving life at a more inspired level. When others ask you to explain how and why, you can venture the opinion that inspired insight does not readily lend itself to intellectual analysis. Rather, understanding can come through a more meditative approach. Intuition and dynamic meditation are twin aspects of this number. A great sense of personal empowerment can come during this year, because we have a chance to view our lives from a higher perspective, and to understand it as energy changing form. Watch your dreams during this cycle and believe that you will understand the deeper meanings behind the symbols. Trust your feelings, and don't overstress the nervous system.

ABOVE: *Dreams are a fruitful source of information and understanding in an Eleven year.*

Twenty-Two — *turning dreams into reality*

Some of the things noted about Number Four will apply here because the reduced number takes on more importance during the relatively short twelve-month cycle of the year. In this case though, Number Four may have a softer feel to it because it carries the sensitivity and vulnerability of the Twenty-Two. It is also an opportunity to start building the dream, to execute the plans that you may feel are really important, but watch out for the effects of over-working. Exhaustion can result, so Number Four may not speak openly of conflicts as readily. Frustration can be internalized, causing stress, so be as compassionate with yourself as you may feel towards others.

Thirty-Three — *lofty ideals*

A tendency to blame yourself for things may be exacerbated during a Thirty-Three year. By all means work towards loftier ideals, but don't let these destabilize relationships that have served you well. There is no need to cast blame if plans do not always work out. The Thirty-Three vibration can rise again to throw up new possibilities of improving the circumstances of your life, whether they are concerned with family or financial issues or with the world at large.

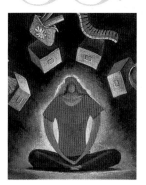

ABOVE: *Idealism is natural during a Thirty-Three year.*

Numbers *in the* Wider world

With numbers we can learn to appreciate more fully the natural and social worlds in which we live.

It is only natural that we should first try to understand the numbers that relate most closely to our own lives. But we can do much more with numbers. We can work with them in a broader social context, and gain insight into our social structures and our position in them. We can relate to numbers emotionally as well as intellectually, and people through the ages have harnessed the complex natural frequencies of sound and expressed them in music. Through numbers we can appreciate more fully the natural world, where they and their vibrations are found as much as in society – the cycle of the four seasons, the repeating shapes of nature in flowers, and the colour spectrum seen in a rainbow are just a few examples.

0

1

2

3

4

5

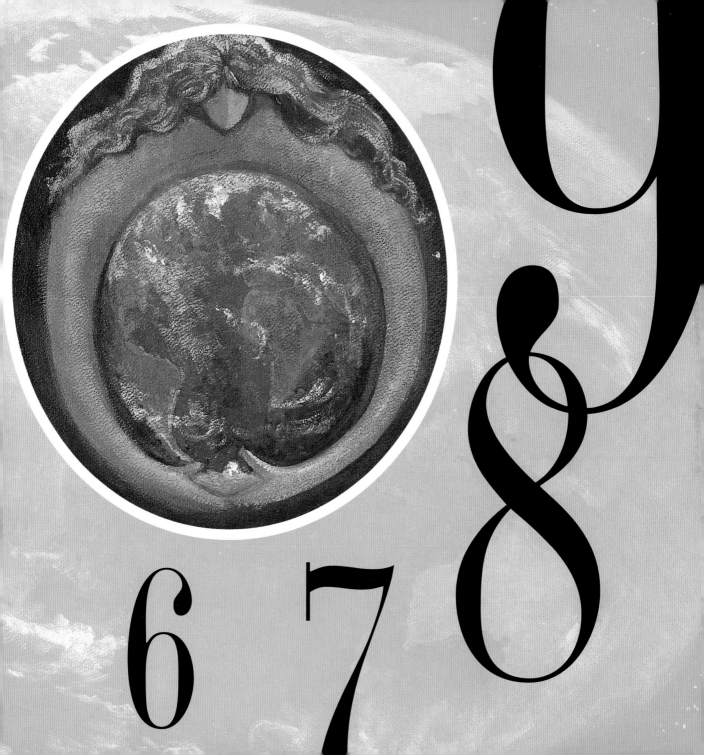

numbers in society

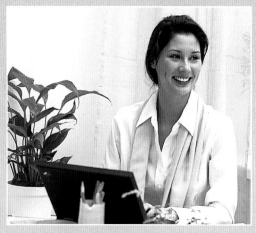

ABOVE: *Our numbers indicate how well we are suited to our work.*

Numbers can broaden and deepen our understanding of ourselves, not simply as isolated individuals but as social beings relating to others one-to-one and in the context of social groups – families, friends, colleagues and the world at large. At work and leisure, we interface with others, unwittingly expressing our numerological characteristics by our choices and behaviours.

NUMEROLOGY IN THE WORKPLACE

The information we get from numbers can be useful in a very practical way in the workplace. For recruitment and personnel management, a numerology profile can show how suited a person is to particular kinds of work or working environments, how they may engage with colleagues and clients, and how they are likely to respond to factors such as stress, deadlines, money, problem-solving or monotonous routine.

This works the other way around too. It is possible to take the numerology profiles of the employees in an organization and match the people to their jobs with some degree of accuracy – without even knowing anything else about them! So on a radio or television station, for instance, those with strong Fives in their profiles are most likely to be the reporters or presenters, in essence the active communicators, while a Seven could be found in the role of producer, working behind the scenes keeping the whole operation running smoothly. It takes all types to make an organization run to its full potential.

NUMBERS, FRIENDS AND LOVERS

Our numbers say a lot about our personality traits, likes and dislikes, so it is easy to see that they can tell us about the people we choose as friends and lovers. So, for example, the outgoing, sometimes hedonistic Five could well be drawn to the independent spirit of the One or the imagination of the Nine, while

We reveal our numbers unwittingly in our behaviour and in the choices we make

a Four could benefit from the uplifting, meditative qualities of a Seven. Of course, it is worth bearing in mind that the qualities that seem attractive at first, such as the sociability of the Five, may not be the ones that suit us in the long run.

CHANGING YOUR NAME

When we begin to use a name other than the one given to us at birth, we immediately project a subtle new vibration and have a different impact on those around us. Although people sometimes think about changing their names in order to give themselves a fresh start, in practice this can be a way of avoiding the spiritual and psychological package that we brought with us into this life.

A change of name for professional purposes can help to demarcate the private and public personas. The particular characteristics with which we came into this world are the ones best suited to helping us maximize our potential in this life and contribute the best we can, but when another name is chosen to fulfil a specific role in public life, such as an actor or singer's stage name or an author's pseudonym, we change our characteristics and create a new potential.

CASE STUDIES

If we look at the numerological values of the original and stage names of two famous entertainers, known to us as Elton John and Marilyn Monroe, we can see how a name can help a person to project a different public image.

Elton John's given name was Reginald Dwight. The Number Six vibration of this name points to issues in his private life that have, in some ways, been worked out in the full gaze of publicity. Here, the Six seeks to internalize and clarify experiences. By assuming the public name Elton John, this performer took on a Number Five vibration, which has provided the stage upon which the Six of his private name has sorted its realities from its illusions. The Five reaches out and puts sexual ambivalence in front of us. This is an aspect of the soul asserting its truth that ultimately the spirit has no identity expressed through gender. The Number Five is also used to channel a strongly individualistic creative drive through music.

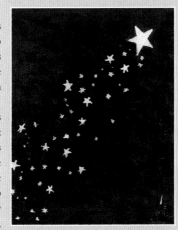

The contrast between the energies of the next pair of names is striking. An analysis of the professional name of the actress **Marilyn Monroe** contains numbers that carry the innocence of fantasy, but the final Six, reduced from 69, questions whether sexuality is a means to a greater love, or another step on the road to decadence.

Her private name, Norma Jean Mortenson, totals up as a Four. However, the vowels, which convey the essence of the person's spirit, reduce to an Eight, while the consonants, denoting the spiritual drive, produce a Five. Here, the Five asks the Eight if she remembers that the inquisitive mind can understand the creative, and sexual, imperative, and allow transformation of her essence to a higher level of awareness. As the public entertainer, Marilyn Monroe, she sought an answer to this question.

ABOVE: *The numerical value of our names determines our star quality and our need to be in the public spotlight.*

numbers in nature

Through self-awareness, people can evolve and rise above unconscious patterns in the natural world. However, such patterns are still instinctive, and firmly rooted in the unconscious. Being "civilized" sets us apart from nature, partly because we feel the need to regulate our instincts to some extent. So it is not surprising to see the proliferation of Nines in a numerological take on this word (three Is as well as the total of the letter values). In the word "civilized", the Nine realizes, to some degree, the understanding and wisdom that has been gained from the cycle. Nature itself carries on unconsciously, and its many patterns can be observed in terms of numbers.

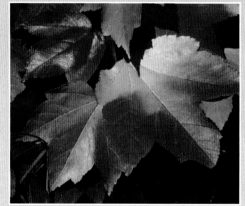

on forever and results in a geometric increase. This reflects an important principle in nature, which is that growth is not purely linear, but builds upon itself. It is self-generating, rather than being dependent on any outside agency to maintain that growth.

An example of how this series is played out in nature can be seen in the number of petals in many wild flowers: far from being random, these often total up to numbers that occur within the Fibonacci series, such as daisies, chamomile and lilies. A geometric increase can be seen in the form of spirals in nature – found in certain shells, or an unfurling fern leaf – which result from growth. The aesthetic appeal of such shapes lies partly in the perfect and simple way that geometries are expressed.

THE FIBONACCI NUMBERS

0 + 1	=	1
1 + 1	=	2
1 + 2	=	3
2 + 3	=	5
3 + 5	=	8
5 + 8	=	13
8 + 13	=	21

This system, dating from the early thirteenth century, describes a pattern of relationships between numbers. It works by repeatedly adding two numbers – always the larger of the figures in the previous addition plus the total of the numbers added in the previous addition – to create a numerical progression.

The series of Fibonacci numbers goes

THREES IN NATURE

In a sense, all life builds on the number Three. We find its most profound expression in the term "trinity", a contraction of "tri-unity", or "Three in One". The Three therefore always carries an imprint of the One, of the original unity, and as the carrier of hope it manifests widely through natural phenomena. Light

ABOVE AND OPPOSITE TOP: *Certain numbers crop up repeatedly in the patterns of nature.*

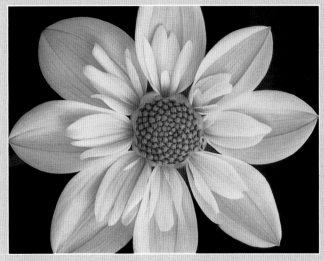

itself – without which there would be no life – is a form of energy that resonates through Number Three. There are three primary colours in the light spectrum – red, yellow and blue-violet – and our perception of colours results from their different wavelengths. The number of colours in light is virtually infinite. All are made from one or more of these three colours, with pure white light consisting of all three in equal quantities and black resulting from an absence of light. In a Number Three profile, light manifests itself as bright ideas and humour.

FOURS IN NATURE

Number Four also provides important frameworks, or building blocks, in nature. The seasons occur in a regular cycle, while the four elements – Earth, Air, Fire and Water – are present everywhere. Both form interlocking systems underpinned by Number Four, in which each season or element is essential.

The elements parallel the subjective states of the human soul. The numbers 1–9 are each associated by the nature of their own energy with one or more of the four elemental energies, and we contain aspects of each of them in our bodies and personalities. The Earth element is expressed in Numbers Four and Eight, which are concerned with holding energy in material form, or regenerating and making more abundant the form that already exists. Air works in the arena of the mind. It is associated with Numbers One and Five, which facilitate change through the generation and communication of new ideas. Fire moves through Numbers Three, Six and Nine, though its expression in the Three is not entirely straightforward as this number carries the passionate aspect of Fire, but expresses it mentally in Air. Water functions in Numbers Two and Seven, where sensitivity is the key. Just as Water pervades the planet, so humanity lives in a sea of emotion.

THE FOUR ELEMENTS

Each of the four elements is associated with particular aspects of the body and human characteristics:

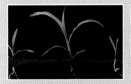 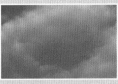 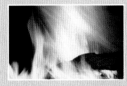 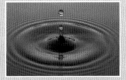

EARTH *body, physical matter, sensation*

AIR *intellect, mind, thought*

FIRE *nervous system, energy, vitality, creativity, movement*

WATER *emotions, feelings, sensitivity*

numbers and music

There is a clear link between music and numbers, and the discovery of this link was the starting point for Pythagoras' development of a theory of numerology. The relationship is captured poetically in his concept of the "music of the spheres" – the idea that music, in the form of sound vibrations, is produced by the motions of the planets and other celestial bodies in our solar system according to the natural laws of harmony.

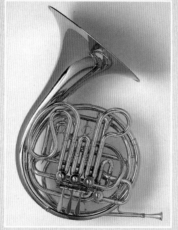

HARMONICS AND PITCH

Every planet has its own primary sound and overtones, in much the same way that if you listen very carefully to a note being played on an instrument such as a violin or flute, you can hear not only the primary note but also a few faint higher notes, called harmonics. Each harmonic is less audible than the previous one, until they are beyond the range of human hearing. The frequency (or the number of vibrations in a unit of time) of these harmonics is always an exact multiple of the frequency of the primary note. The intervals between the harmonics are not equal but become progressively closer; however, the ratio of the frequencies to each other is always exactly the same. It makes no difference which note is played; the harmonics always resonate in the same ratio. If you hear an instrument or an orchestra that sounds out of tune, it is because these ratios between the notes are not exact. Emotionally we respond to this strongly as we feel the disharmony in the relationships between the sounds.

As well as having harmonics, the primary note of each celestial body has a unique pitch, or frequency. Just as the harmonics of a note resonate in a fixed, measurable relationship to each other, the intervals between the notes of a major scale are also in a fixed ratio, the top note in the scale being exactly double the frequency of the bottom note. The progressive sequence of celestial frequencies is similar to the eight-note diatonic scale of Western music. It is no coincidence that this scale brought the influence of Number Eight into greater prominence in our civilization, and with it the rigour and responsibilities of this number.

THE TONE OF YOUR LIFE

The philosopher and thinker G. I. Gurdjieff developed the idea that life moves in octaves, providing another way of thinking of the cyclical nature of existence. To try out this idea, sing or hum the notes of a scale, thinking of each note as a different year of your life as you progress slowly upwards. Note any impressions that come to mind.

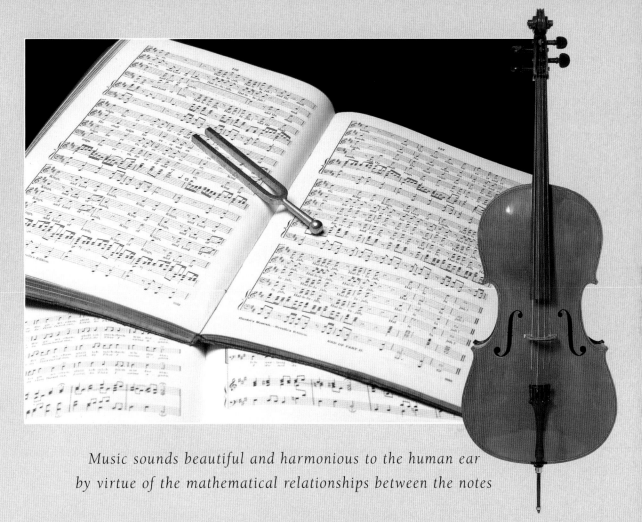

Music sounds beautiful and harmonious to the human ear by virtue of the mathematical relationships between the notes

HARMONY

The relationships between different notes sounding together are the building blocks of harmony. The three-note chord or triad is the building block of music: if each note of a single triad is used as the building block for a new triad, five such combinations will generate every note of the scale. Harmonies give complexity to music and evoke feelings in us; the discords of innovation become the sweet harmonies of the future as our sensibilities evolve.

EXPRESSING ENERGY THROUGH MUSIC

A parallel can be drawn between the Western musical scale and the cycles of One to Nine (whether natural cycles or the progressions of consciousness): both are movement of energy, expressed through sequences of numbers. Not only is our passage through life symbolized by the numbers, but the energy moves through those numbers and is changed by them in a measurable geometric pattern.

ABOVE: *The single note of the tuning fork is always the same; this simple instrument provides the basis of a well-tuned orchestra.*
OPPOSITE: *The precise positioning of the keys of brass and wind instruments is calculated mathematically.*

visualization and dreaming

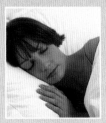

There are various ways of understanding the meanings of numbers – such as by looking at their unique energies, and their association with your name and birth date. The story of the cycle of numbers is illustrated by people's lives and unfolds through the different stages of life, at various age points, and through the personal year cycles. With this understanding, you can start drawing a kind of route map of your own life, of what seems to make you tick as an individual, and how you interact with the world around you.

But intellectual understanding will help only so far. To get the most out of the numbers, it helps if we look at them in a more open or intuitive way. Ideally, we should approach the numbers afresh every time, avoiding the preconceived ideas we may have about them, and listen to what they are trying to tell us.

For most of us this may well seem difficult to achieve at first. Two useful ways to develop a more open, intuitive and non-judgemental way of listening to the numbers are visualization and dreaming. With these techniques we use the subjective side of our natures to access what we already know unconsciously.

VISUALIZATION

For many people, an ideal time to practise visualization is at night shortly before going to sleep, although you can make use of any other quiet time. Sit comfortably in loose-fitting clothes, close your eyes, and become aware of your breathing. It should be slow and purposeful, but not forced, and not too deep.

With your eyes still closed gaze into the black space between the eyebrows, known by some as the third eye, or ajna. Picture a number between one and nine. Let us suppose that you are looking at Number Eight. First, just look at the number, then move towards it inwardly, step inside it if you want. Throughout this exercise, remember that your purpose in doing it is to obtain further insight into the energy of the number.

After five minutes or so, come back to waking awareness. Make a written note of any impressions that came to you during the session. If you repeat the exercise over a number of weeks, your understanding of the numbers will broaden and deepen. You can carry out the same procedure with each of the numbers between one and nine.

DREAMING

This is an extension of visualization and harnesses the power of suggestion over your unconscious. Just before dropping off to sleep, place your attention lightly upon a number that you have chosen, and hold it there gently as you fall into slumber. At the same time, keep in your mind the idea that you will, upon waking, find you have been given some new insight into the number.

When you wake up, make a few notes of anything that you can remember from your dream. Try this perhaps once a week for a month and keep a note of any results obtained.

ABOVE LEFT AND OPPOSITE: *Sleep is a productive time for our unconscious minds, and we can harness the power of our dreams to develop our intuitive understanding of numbers.*

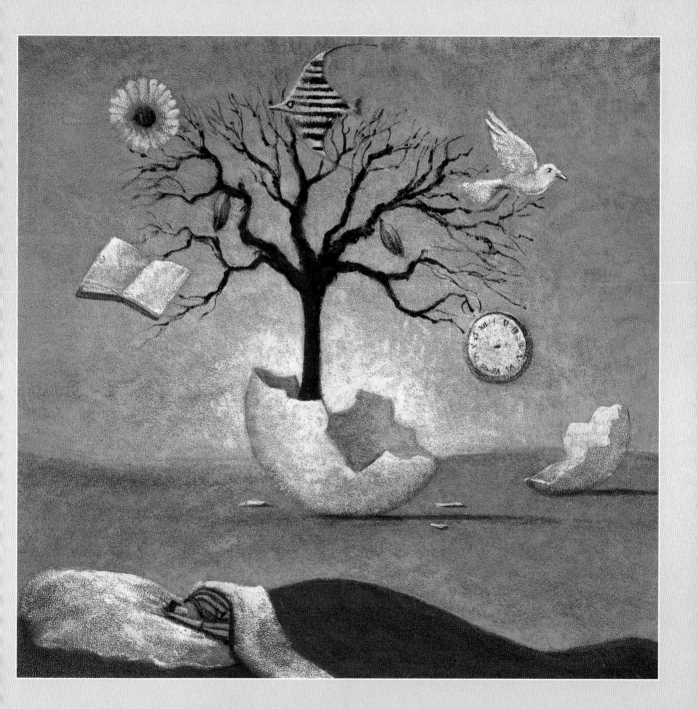

numbers in esoteric traditions

Awareness of the relationships between different energies, and of the significance of numbers in various arcane arts, gives us useful layers of meaning to work with when we are trying to understand how we function and develop in our lives.

Esoteric traditions differ in their methods and underlying beliefs, but they all investigate the mysteries of the universe. Often they have arisen from similar social and historical contexts or have built on each other to develop into new systems. As well as being tools for gaining personal insight, they are sometimes used for divination, by extrapolating future events from existing trends or patterns. Three such systems that have strong links with numerology are Tarot, the Kabbalah and astrology. All three work with sequences or cycles and show a symbolic progression from birth and action in the first stage to death and completion in the last.

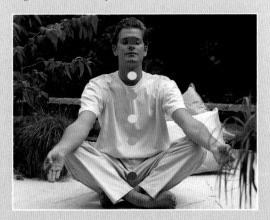

TAROT, THE KABBALAH AND ASTROLOGY

The cards in the Tarot pack are grouped and numbered to provide several layers of significance: the 22 picture cards of the major arcana represent personal qualities or archetypes, or stages on a spiritual journey, while the numbered cards of the minor arcana depict the different phases of that journey seen through the four elements, Fire, Air, Earth and Water.

The Tree of Life of the Kabbalah maps our developmental journey through life diagrammatically; the 22 paths on this diagram directly parallel the Tarot's major arcana.

The influences of the planets, sun and moon, along with the related attributes of the 12 signs of the Zodiac, are among the fundamental tools of astrology. They too can contribute to your

Numbers provide extra layers of meaning and interpretation in the arcane arts

understanding of numerology if you relate the astrology cycles to the cycles of the numbers, and the meanings contained in a numerology reading might correlate with your astrological chart, depending on the level of the reading given.

COLOUR ENERGY AND OUR CHAKRAS

We can also find other energy forms resonating with the numbers. Colours, which are manifestations of light energy being absorbed and reflected, have their own vibrations;

LEFT: *Each chakra reverberates to a different energy vibration.*

THE KABBALAH

Passed down the generations in secret and by word of mouth, the Kabbalah has evolved over many centuries. This body of teachings is central to the Jewish mystical tradition. In this tradition, two ways of investigating and explaining the mysteries of our spiritual life and our relationship with God are *gematria* and the Tree of Life.

In the Middle Ages, Kabbalists developed gematria, a numerical interpretation of the Hebrew Scriptures which has similarities with Pythagorean numerology. The 22 Hebrew letters each have a numeric value and a symbolic meaning as well as representing a phonetic sound. Working with these values and symbols, words of equal numeric value can be correlated to find deeper layers of meaning.

A key visual and conceptual tool used in working with the Kabbalah is the Tree of Life, which consists of 10 numbered spheres, linked by 22 paths, plus

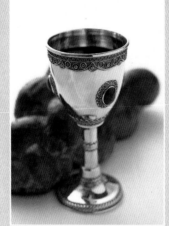

one unnumbered sphere. Each sphere is named and represents a personal or spiritual quality, and there are clear parallels between these qualities and the meanings of the numbers 0–9 in numerology. The connecting paths are assigned a numerical value and are also indicated by the 22 richly symbolic letters of the Hebrew alphabet.

Moving up the Tree represents the progression through three levels of consciousness, from basic earthly qualities of body and personality (senses, subconscious, intellect and feeling) through the soul (ego, individual will and individual love) to the spirit (spiritual love, spiritual will and pure spirit). The spheres are also thought to have a dark side and a light side, seen as negative and positive aspects, while the left and right sides contain the polarities of masculine and feminine. Constant inter-relationship between the spheres brings about evolution and growth further up the Tree.

because of this we can relate each number, with its associated moods and personalities, to a colour or range of colours. Countless generations have developed symbolic associations with the different colours, while the colours we naturally choose to work with – especially in our clothes and décor – are a means of self-expression. You may find that you have a connection with the colours of your dominant numbers.

Similarly, each of the numbers 1–9 also has a particular relationship with one or more of the seven chakras – the energy centres of the body which govern a person's spiritual, mental and physical wellbeing, and which are in themselves associated with particular colours.

ABOVE: *Every culture has its own numerical energy vibration.*

next steps

Like other esoteric arts, numerology is an extremely complex system that has many variations and can be worked with at many levels and degrees of detail. Two approaches to take if you wish to build on the foundations you have laid so far are to broaden your investigations into how numerology can be used in your life, and to deepen your understanding of numerology by finding out more about the subtleties of this discipline.

BROADENING YOUR INVESTIGATIONS

Even at a relatively basic level, the information and insights provided by numerology can be used to look beyond our name and birth date at other numbers in our lives. Our

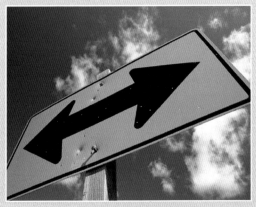

ABOVE: *Numbers can help us to understand the choices we have.*
OPPOSITE: *Even our house number can say something about our life choices.*

address, telephone number, and driving licence number, for instance, all resonate with us in some way. If your house number coincides with your Life Path Number, for instance, an energy alignment may occur which could help you to fulfil your potential more easily, though it could also mean that negative traits of that number are accentuated as well.

Becoming aware of ourselves and of the significance of the numbers can help us to live in harmony with our lives and make the most of situations. Just as you can derive a Personal Year Number from your birth date and the year of your most recent birthday, you can also find your Personal Month Number by adding your Personal Year Number to the number of the current month, and your Personal Day Number by adding the Personal Month Number to the current day of the month. Each day and month has a particular vibration for an individual, and this information can help to provide you with a focus for the way you approach your life during these periods of time.

Numbers give us insights into the wider context of our world too. The letters of every word have a numeric value, and give us a deeper understanding of the resonance of that word. Translating letters into numbers enables us to get a sense of the energy of any word. We saw earlier how the word "civilized" resonates with its numerological value, Number Nine. Taking this further, we can even look at just part of a word, for instance in the suffix "-logy", which indicates science, theory and discourse; the values of the letters – 3, 6, 7, and 7 – reduce to Five, the number that relates to reaching understanding through investigation and experience.

Once you have a feeling for the general qualities of the numbers, you can try to get a deeper understanding of the numbers by learning to appreciate their more subtle qualities. You can also investigate the complexities of the various approaches to numerology.

The birth date can be accessed in several ways. For instance, in one method, some of the numbers of this date are used to reveal past life factors that may be affecting a person in the present cycle of existence. Another specifically alchemical approach to numerology includes an in-depth examination of age and spiritual maturity, and attempts to understand why the process of spiritual growth can get blocked or slowed down.

Your name, as we have seen, can be expressed in numbers to reveal patterns of behaviour and spiritual motivation which, in part, go back over generations. This concept can be taken

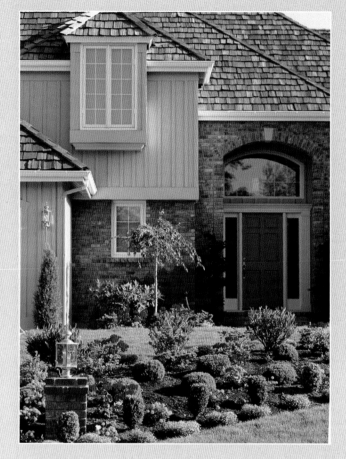

Numerology can be understood at many levels, giving us access to deeper insights

further by focusing on individual letters and numbers within a name. The presence or absence of certain numbers in your name can tell us about the strong and weak aspects of your personal make-up, while the vowels and consonants are often treated separately: in a literal sense the vowels carry the sound of a name, while the consonants anchor the sound in the

material world. Translated into numerology terms then, the vowels carry the essence of your spirit, and the consonants give form to your spiritual drive. In the example shown, the spirited sociability of the Five found in the vowels is grounded in the steady Four of the name's consonants.

As you investigate numerology more fully, you may find inconsistencies between different approaches. Don't be disheartened by this: listen to your own intuitive feelings to discover which approaches make most sense to you, and which ones best address the issues you wish to work with in your life. Often information that seems to be at odds with another source is in reality merely providing a different perspective on the same idea.

1			5		5			7	5			23/5
A	N	N	H	E	L	E	N	M	Y	E	R	S
5	5	8		3		5	4		9	1		40/4
												63/9

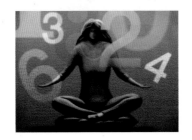

index

FURTHER INFORMATION

If you would like to discover more about numerology, a good source of information and contacts is the Association Internationale de Numerologues. Membership of the A.I.N. is open to anyone who is interested in numerology, and benefits of membership include a regular newsletter. The association can also provide contact details of qualified numerologists who are available to do readings.

    To go more deeply into numerology, introductory and advanced courses can be taken at The Connaissance School of Numerology.

The Association and the School are both located at:

The Cave Shop
8 Melbourn Street
Royston
Hertfordshire, SG8 7BZ
UK
www.numerology.org.uk

The website contains much useful information on numerology, together with notices of forthcoming events.